I hope you are having a great day, because [...] level is up and I feel like I can accomplish anything I set my mind to. I have lost ten pounds in the past ten days! —Helen Allen

When I started the detox, I felt hopeless, at my all-time high weight of 270 pounds. This morning, Day 10, I weigh under 253 pounds!! I feel so great. I'm sleeping soundly, have less anxiety, feel hopeful, and my knee is hurting so much less. I'm very excited to keep going. Getting such quick results, learning how to cook real food, and feeling alert have given me the confidence I've needed to move forward and stay with this style of eating and living. —Patricia Swanson

This has completely changed my life! I can't believe how much weight I have lost in such a short amount of time. But more importantly, I feel so much better. I have suffered for years from insomnia…to finally be able to hit the pillow and go to sleep…priceless! —Lauren Creekmur

It really did work. I lost eleven pounds, and my blood sugar is down over forty points. I never even knew it was high. My blood pressure— which I also never knew was elevated—has returned to normal. I think this was a gift that came at a time I really needed it, and didn't quite know how much. —Martha Broyles

Possibly the best part for me as a former sugar addict: no sugar for twelve days! I'm now convinced that this and even greater health changes are possible for anyone when we make the powerful choices that support our body, mind, and spirit in being well. —Jodi Briden

I have been struggling with acne for the past year, and amazingly over the last ten days my skin has almost completely cleared up. I couldn't be happier with the way I look and feel. —Sara Fleischhauer

Although I knew prior to the start of the program that I had hypertension, I didn't get the results of my blood test until Day 4, when I found out I have type 2 diabetes. My fasting glucose level was 152. Since this diet, my fasting glucose levels have been between 98 and 110. I'm totally convinced this diet is going to help me regain my health, energy, and passion for life that I had felt slipping away.   —David Swan

I am calmer and thinner. I have another thirty-five pounds to lose and now have the confidence that it can be done. I used to be an above-average fit person...I was very much in self-loathing about that. Not today. I can't thank you enough.   —Jim Portz

I am more clear-headed than I have been in a long time. I did lose weight, but I am more excited about how great I feel.

—Jennifer Lawrence

A coworker commented on Day 6 that I looked different. I asked what he meant by "different" and he replied, "You're glowing." That's just what I needed to hear to know the diet was truly making a difference.

—Fay Switsky

I have been struggling for years with depression. I used to be the one with boundless energy and a smile on my face, but as time went by, I saw that person less and less. When I was given the chance to try the 10-Day Detox, I knew this was my chance. The end result was ten pounds lost, but more importantly, I began to find the old me. The person with the winning outlook began to reappear and the fog began to lift. Dr. Hyman used the word "vitality"...that is a great word to explain what I have been given back through this opportunity.

—Charlene Wynant

THE **BLOOD SUGAR SOLUTION**

10-DAY
DETOX
DIET

THE **BLOOD SUGAR SOLUTION**

10-DAY DETOX DIET

Activate Your Body's Natural Ability to Burn Fat and Lose Weight Fast

Mark Hyman

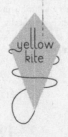

For my children, Rachel and Misha

First published the USA in 2014 by Little, Brown and Company
Hachette Book Group Inc

First published in Great Britain in 2014 by Hodder & Stoughton
An Hachette UK company

This edition published in 2016 by Yellow Kite Books
An imprint of Hodder & Stoughton
An Hachette UK company

4

A CIP catalogue record for this title is available from the British Library.

Paperback ISBN 978 1 444 75155 0
Ebook ISBN 978 1 444 75154 3

Printed and bound by Clays Ltd, St Ives plc

Hodder & Stoughton policy is to use papers that are natural, renewable and recyclable products and made from wood grown in sustainable forests. The logging and manufacturing processes are expected to conform to the environmental regulations of the country of origin.

This book is intended to supplement, not replace, the advice of a trained health professional. If you know or suspect that you have a health problem, you should consult a health professional. The author and publisher specifically disclaim any liability, loss, or risk, personal or otherwise, that is incurred as a consequence, directly or indirectly, of the use and application of any of the contents of this book.

Hodder & Stoughton Ltd
Carmelite House
50 Victoria Embankment
London EC4Y 0DZ

www.hodder.co.uk

Contents

Contents

PART V

THE TRANSITION PHASE

PART VI

IT'S BIGGER THAN US

PART VII

THE 10-DAY DETOX MEAL PLAN AND RECIPES

An Invitation

Janet, a forty-eight-year-old woman, came to see me after struggling half her life with her weight and health. She was always busy taking care of things, but never herself. Janet had gained 100 pounds (45 kg) since high school and, despite trying many diets and working with different nutritionists over the years, she could not get ahold of her eating habits. Instead, they had control over her. Her father had type 2 diabetes, and she had experienced gestational diabetes during her pregnancies, so she knew she was at risk for the disease. Highly intelligent and successful in every area of her life, Janet was failing miserably in her health. She knew she needed to do something about it—and fast.

Janet ate well...or so she thought. For breakfast, she would have whole-wheat toast and coffee with fat-free milk, unknowingly starting her day with two of the foods that can cause the most inflammation—gluten and dairy. At lunch, she would eat whatever her office staff ordered in: Thai, Chinese, "healthy stuff" like rice and noodles (just sugar in a different form). In the afternoon she would crave sugar, and because her workplace was full of candy and junk food, she would eat it—usually steadily throughout the afternoon. Dinners were generally good, she thought, with fish, broccoli, corn, and potatoes. Unfortunately, the "large" fish she was choosing, such as tuna and swordfish, were loaded with mercury, which creates toxicity and inflammation in the body, leading to more weight gain. She enjoyed a few glasses of wine with dinner because she'd heard wine was good for you. After dinner, she craved sweets and, like many people, went after cake and cookies with seemingly no "off" switch. She then felt guilty and berated herself for "ruining" her diet with junk and sweets. As hard as she tried to will herself to stop, she couldn't. She was a prisoner of food addiction.

Janet worked out for forty minutes about four days a week on the elliptical machine and did strength training twice a week. This was good, but I was worried about her. Her lab tests showed a terrible cholesterol profile, with high triglycerides, low HDL (good cholesterol), and high LDL (bad cholesterol); a blood sugar of 107 fasting (pre-diabetes); and a high level of blood inflammation with a C-reactive protein of 8.8 (normal is less than 1).

All this did not bode well for her. With further testing, we found she had super-high insulin levels. A normal fasting level is 5 to 10; hers was 27. After a sugar drink, a normal level is 20 to 30; hers was 231! Here was the key component of Janet's weight struggles: **Insulin makes you hungry and makes you store belly fat.** Janet's body was suffering not because of too much food or too little exercise, but because what she was eating and how she was living were disrupting her insulin levels. Her hormones were running the show.

We ran the test that measures average blood sugar over six weeks, called hemoglobin A1c, and it turned out she was a type 2 diabetic and didn't know it (anything over 5.9 is diabetes, and over 5.5 is considered at-risk; Janet's score was 6.5). Plus, her blood mercury was very high at 23 (normal is less than 3) because of all the large fish she was eating.

We put her on the Blood Sugar Solution 10-Day Detox Diet, and after the first few days, her cravings disappeared and her weight started dropping off. In just ten days she lost eleven pounds (5 kg). We got her off the big fish and onto eating small fish; got her off the processed bread, noodles, and rice and onto whole, real, fresh food; and got her doing a bit more self-nurturing. To her surprise, the powerful drive to consume sugar vanished, and she could easily walk right past the treats in her office that used to call out to her. Her evenings were now about relaxing and enjoying time with her family, rather than snacking and guilt.

After three months on the detox, she had lost a total of forty-four pounds (20 kg) and was still dropping. Her test scores normalized, showing a normal hemoglobin A1c (5.3). No more diabetes. Her inflammation and cholesterol levels also came down without any medication. The numbers on the scale continued to go down as her health soared.

Janet tells me that she uses the tools she learned on the Blood Sugar Solution 10-Day Detox Diet to listen to her body and give it—and herself—the care she needs. Her cravings are a thing of the past. Though still surprised she was able to do it so easily, Janet finally feels at peace with her relationship with food and her now-healthy body.

I want to invite you to take a journey with me toward health, but first let me tell you why.

I have an extraordinary job. I have the privilege of caring for people, of being of service every day, of using my mind, experience, and knowledge to guide my patients toward greater well-being. Medical science has advanced faster than medical practice, which is often twenty to thirty years out of date. Yet there is a movement to change that. As the chairman of the board of directors of the Institute for Functional Medicine, I am part of the transformation of medical education and practice that will change our notions and treatment of disease completely. In fact, most medicine of the future will not be about directly treating illness. Instead, it will be about creating health. Disease simply goes away as a side effect of creating health.

And here's another side effect: *automatic weight loss*. In fact, I never tell my patients to lose weight. I simply help them restore health, and the magic of biology does the rest. Your goal in picking up this book may be to lose weight; my goal is to get you healthy. Either way, we both win.

I treat patients one by one in my office, and in a year can see only so many people, yet millions and millions suffer needlessly, which is why I teach, write books, and speak around the world. I want to provide a clear solution for people to practice self-care. I want to teach the simple principles and lay out the "goof-proof" steps to optimal health and sustainable weight loss.

The Blood Sugar Solution 10-Day Detox Diet is a chance to engage in a transformative experience that will show you the power you have to feel better—not in weeks or months, but *now.* This is a ten-day reboot for your entire system. It will reset your biology and metabolism, enabling you to reverse chronic symptoms and effortlessly break free of your cravings and lose weight. This is a way to quickly and profoundly change your life just by changing a few basic things: what you eat, how you move, how you rest, how you recharge, and how you connect.

Most doctors (and a great many other people) don't believe that you can achieve the radical health and weight transformation you're seeking in just the span of a few days. But I do. That is why I created a trial program of the Blood Sugar Solution 10-Day Detox Diet in early 2013. I wanted to prove to people just how quickly and easily they could lose the weight that plagued them and how close they really were to feeling better than they had in years.

Over six hundred people in our online community signed up for the program. My goal was to help them experience firsthand the restorative magic of their own biology, and to reconnect with their natural state of vitality. It's one thing to hear in the abstract that something like this is possible, and another to see and feel the results for yourself. I understood that, at first, many would be skeptical, so I made them a bold promise: *Just give me ten days and your life will never be the same.*

Not only did the trial participants lose dramatic amounts of weight (4,089 pounds/1,855 kg total) and inches off their waists, but their average blood sugar dropped twenty points and their blood pressure went down almost ten points. Their brain fog evaporated and chronic symptoms disappeared. Many wrote in to tell me they looked and felt better than they ever could have imagined (you'll hear much more from these participants throughout the book). Best of all, they emerged from the prison of addiction without cravings, reclaiming control of their appetite, mood, and brain chemistry. And this all happened in just the first ten days!

If these six hundred people could have these kinds of results, you can, too. I will make you the same promise I made them, with the same goal of allowing you to witness your body's own amazing healing potential. If you follow the program, you'll experience for yourself just how easy and attainable this really is. Stick with it for ten days, and I'm guessing you will want to incorporate many components of the program in your life for the longer term. And that's fine, because really, this is a road map for life, for whenever you want to find your way back to your natural state of health, energy, and well-being.

Naturally, my hope is that you continue to progress on this path. But if *The Blood Sugar Solution 10-Day Detox Diet* does nothing else but show you that you CAN change your life...that you CAN eat in a way that creates effortless appetite control and curbs cravings...that you CAN lose weight and keep it off...that you CAN get your diabetes and blood pressure under control, then I've done what I set out to do.

THE BLOOD SUGAR SOLUTION

10-DAY
DETOX
DIET

Introduction

Are you ready for a total body revolution?

Welcome to the Blood Sugar Solution 10-Day Detox Diet!

In my book *The Blood Sugar Solution,* I shared my proven six-week plan for preventing, treating, and even reversing diabetes and pre-diabetes. Millions of people were amazed as they fixed their life-threatening blood sugar problems. At the same time, the program kicked their metabolism into high gear and they easily lost stubborn belly fat.

Now, for the first time, I have created a fast-track plan that will enable you to shed upwards of ten pounds (5 kg) and radically reboot your entire system *in just ten short days.* With the right combination of powerful foods and practices, we're going to stop your fat-storage hormone in its tracks, cool off the inflammation that contributes to weight gain, and upgrade your detox pathways. You'll lose weight with astonishing speed and ease—and keep it off using these lifelong tools and strategies for maximum success.

With the 10-Day Detox Diet, we're going to get rid of more than just unwanted pounds. This is your chance to heal your body *on every level.* Yes, you will drop pounds, but you will also find that your energy, sleep, and mood improve, that chronic problems including joint pain, digestive problems, autoimmune disease, headaches, memory problems and brain fog, sinus and allergy issues, even acne, eczema, and psoriasis will get better or disappear entirely. Your sexual desire and function may even improve.

Why is that the case? Because **what makes you sick also makes you fat, and what makes you fat makes you sick.** Let me explain. Health is a state of balance, and disease is a state of imbalance. When

3

you begin to put on weight, especially lethal belly fat, your biology shifts out of balance, veering into the unstable and unhealthy territory of disease—which in turn makes you fatter.

One point that a growing number of doctors like me agree upon is that the whole idea of "disease" itself is wrong. We recognize disease only when we reach a certain level of symptoms or results on our blood tests. For example, if your blood sugar is 98 mg/dl, it is normal, but if it is 101 mg/dl, you have pre-diabetes. If your blood sugar is 124 mg/dl, you have pre-diabetes, but if it is 127 mg/dl, you have type 2 diabetes. This is absurd.

Imbalance occurs along a continuum, and the farther along that continuum you are, the more problems you have. Many people have whole collections of symptoms, conditions, and diseases—obesity, diabetes, high blood pressure, high cholesterol, arthritis, depression, reflux, irritable bowel, autoimmune disease, asthma, and more.

I call myself a "wholistic" doctor, because I take care of patients with a "whole list" of symptoms. In treating such patients, I've often found that their health complaints are not really separate problems. They are all related and driven by a few common root causes: what they eat; how much they move, rest, connect; and how toxic they are.

What we have found in functional medicine is that everything is connected—this is called *systems medicine*. Your body is one integrated, interdependent system. That is why, when you get to the root cause or causes, so many often-related symptoms go away without having to be addressed individually. It is medicine by cause, not by symptom. It is medicine of your whole system, not by geography or where the symptoms are located in your body. By connecting the dots, we can find a clear path to health and wellness.

Here's how this all ties in with weight: The factors that cause your symptoms are the very same factors that cause weight gain, pre-diabetes, and diabetes. Those factors include inflammation, hormonal imbalance, toxicity, and more. But remember, it's all connected, so your excess weight problems very likely share many of the same root causes as your other health complaints. As you follow the program, you'll come to understand how the ways you eat, move, relax, live, and think can quickly create either an environment of healing or an environment of toxicity within your body, and set the stage for weight gain or weight loss.

It comes down to this: If you're toxic, it makes you sick and fat. That is why I want you to take the Toxicity Questionnaire below, both before beginning the 10-Day Detox Diet, and again after you've completed the ten days. It will give you a baseline for your existing symptoms, which are indications of being toxic and inflamed. But even more, it will help you connect the dots and see the interconnections in your body, and see for yourself how, after just ten days, you can enjoy such a dramatic reduction in symptoms and problems.

Those who did the 10-Day Detox Diet experienced a 62 percent reduction in their symptoms. Think about that: There is no drug on the planet that can reduce all these symptoms in just ten days! But if you treat your whole system, rather than individual symptoms, extraordinary healing and weight loss can occur.

ARE YOU SICK? THE TOXICITY QUESTIONNAIRE

For the "before" part of the questionnaire, rate each of the following symptoms based upon your health profile for the past thirty days. You'll take this quiz again after your 10-Day Detox, but it's especially important that you take the time to complete and score it now, before you embark on the program. Without that baseline score, ten days from now you may have a hard time believing just how different your "after" results really are.

Point Scale
0 = Never or almost never have the symptom
1 = Occasionally have it, effect is not severe
2 = Occasionally have it, effect is severe
3 = Frequently have it, effect is not severe
4 = Frequently have it, effect is severe

Digestive Tract

1	Nausea or vomiting
2	Diarrhea
0	Constipation
4	Bloated feeling
3	Belching, or passing gas
4	Heartburn
1	Intestinal, stomach pain

Total before 15

Total after _____

Ears

0	Itchy ears
1	Earaches, ear infections
0	Drainage from ear
4	Ringing in ears, hearing loss

Total before 5

Total after _____

Emotions

2	Mood swings
4	Anxiety, fear, or nervousness
1	Anger, irritability, or aggressiveness
1	Depression

Total before 8

Total after _____

Energy/Activity

4	Fatigue, sluggishness
3	Apathy, lethargy
1	Hyperactivity
2	Restlessness

Total before 10

Total after _____

Eyes

4	Watery or itchy eyes
1	Swollen, reddened, or sticky eyelids
1	Bags or dark circles under eyes
1	Blurred or tunnel vision (does not include near- or farsightedness)

Total before 7

Total after _____

Head

4	Headaches
0	Faintness
1	Dizziness
0	Insomnia

Total before 5

Total after _____

Heart

3	Irregular or skipped heartbeat
3	Rapid or pounding heartbeat
1	Chest pain

Total before 7

Total after _____

Joints/Muscles

3	Pain or aches in joints
4	Arthritis
1	Stiffness or limitation of movement
1	Pain or aches in muscles
1	Feeling of weakness or tiredness

Total before 10

Total after _____

Lungs

0	Chest congestion
0	Asthma, bronchitis
3	Shortness of breath
1	Difficulty breathing

Total before 4

Total after _____

Mind

___4___ Poor memory
___3___ Confusion, poor comprehension
___3___ Poor concentration
___1___ Poor physical coordination
___4___ Difficulty in making decisions
___1___ Stuttering or stammering
___0___ Slurred speech
___0___ Learning disabilities
Total before ___16___
Total after _____

Mouth/Throat

___1___ Chronic coughing
___0___ Gagging, frequent need to clear throat
___3___ Sore throat, hoarseness, loss of voice
___0___ Swollen or discolored tongue, gums, or lips
___3___ Canker sores
Total before ___7___
Total after _____

Nose

___3___ Stuffy nose
___1___ Sinus problems
___3___ Hay fever
___1___ Excessive mucus formation
___0___ Sneezing attacks
Total before ___8___
Total after _____

Skin

___1___ Acne
___2___ Hives, rashes, or dry skin
___3___ Hair loss
___2___ Flushing or hot flushes
___1___ Excessive sweating
Total before ___9___
Total after _____

Weight

___1___ Binge eating/drinking
___4___ Craving certain foods
___4___ Excessive weight
___1___ Compulsive eating
___1___ Water retention
___0___ Underweight
Total before ___11___
Total after _____

Other

___1___ Frequent illness
___1___ Frequent or urgent urination
___1___ Genital itch or discharge
Total before ___3___
Total after _____

GRAND TOTAL BEFORE ___125___

GRAND TOTAL AFTER _____

Key to Questionnaire

Optimal health: less than 10
Mild toxicity: 10 to 50
Moderate toxicity: 50 to 100
Severe toxicity: over 100

WHY DETOX?

If you are overweight, there's a very good chance that you're a food addict. But let me stop right there and tell you that I'm not blaming you. You are not gluttonous, nor weak-willed, nor any other self-recriminating belief you may have about yourself and your relationship to food. Your hormones, taste buds, and brain chemistry have been hijacked by the food industry. Not metaphorically, but biologically. You are hooked—a junkie mainlining some of the worst, deadliest drugs on the planet: sugar and anything that turns to sugar in your body. That's why you're here to detox.

The $1-trillion industrial food system is the biggest drug dealer around, responsible for contributing to tens of millions of deaths every year and siphoning trillions of dollars from our global economy through the loss of human and natural capital. I realize this sounds extreme and overstated, but hear me out. Once you understand the forces at play in food addiction, you will never think the same way again about Snapple, Diet Coke, and processed snacks, cookies, and cake.

We need to acknowledge our addiction, face it, and address it head-on, both as individuals and as a society. We need a big solution that reaches deep into what is offered in our supermarkets, restaurants, schools, and workplaces. We need a solution that addresses the policy roots in agriculture, food marketing, dietary recommendations, and the way doctors are trained to diagnose and treat patients.

But first, you need to take back your own health. And I'm here to help you do exactly that.

In order to break free from these addictive substances and reprogram your biology, you need to detox from the druglike foods and beverages you've been hooked on. We now know—because it has been scientifically proven—that sugar is more powerfully addictive than alcohol, cocaine, or even heroin (and if you're thinking about going for diet soda instead, take note: Artificial sweeteners may be more addictive than regular sugar). When we treat alcoholics or cocaine addicts, we don't say "Practice moderation" and advise them to cut down to just one drink or one line of cocaine a day. We know they must clear the brain and body of these powerful drugs completely, ideally through a well-designed program that supports the detox process.

That's precisely what we're going to do here. In just ten days, you'll have a whole new level of clarity, both physically and mentally. You'll know with certainty that you *can* regain control, feel good, and change your life forever.

But what if you're trying this diet just to lose some weight and make good on your New Year's resolution? That's fine. We all want to look good! The magic in the 10-Day Detox Diet is that you'll end up not just *looking* fantastic, but feeling fantastic, too—quite possibly better than you ever imagined.

Just to be clear, though, the Blood Sugar Solution 10-Day Detox Diet is not a magic cure or a gimmicky weight loss scheme. It is a comprehensive, science-based approach to ending food addiction and creating rapid, safe weight loss and long-term optimal health. It is for anyone who wants to experience what true wellness feels like, and for most people, that realization is just ten days away.

Again, I realize that you may not believe all this is possible. And you don't have to. All you have to do is give it a try and see for yourself how quickly the body heals and sheds pounds when it is getting what it really needs.

Most of my patients say, "Dr. Hyman, I didn't know I was feeling so bad until I started feeling so good." After doing the Blood Sugar Solution 10-Day Detox Diet, you'll likely be saying the same thing.

How to Use This Book

Let me give you a quick overview of the book.

In **Part I,** I explain the nature of food addiction and how our biology has been held hostage by the food industry. I will help you fix your "fat thinking," dispelling the myths that keep you fat and sick and helping you find a path to food freedom.

In **Part II,** I explain how the program works, including what you'll do, what you'll eat, who you will have on your side, how you will track your results, and how you can get rid of the bad stuff and add in the good stuff to create effortless healing and weight loss.

In **Part III,** I'll take you through the Prep Phase, during which you will do six simple things to get ready: detox your kitchen; gather your supplies; taper off caffeine, alcohol, and sugar; align your mind and intentions; measure yourself; and connect with the Blood Sugar Solution 10-Day Detox Diet online community to get the support you need.

In **Part IV,** I'll give you a step-by-step, goof-proof plan for each of the ten days. You will receive your daily schedule and learn about each component of your daily routine, which, when done synergistically, will generate powerful healing and weight loss. Each day has a unique focus and a journaling exercise related to the changes you will be experiencing. These are designed to take you deeper into the detox process and help you transform lifelong bad habits into conditions for lifelong success.

In **Part V,** you will learn how to gently and safely transition into a long-term plan personalized specifically for your needs.

In **Part VI,** I'll explain the power of giving back. You'll find out how you can be part of the larger solution to the health and obesity crisis affecting our families, our communities, our nation, other nations, and even the planet. You'll also discover how becoming a part of this new, empowering health revolution can benefit you directly. Part VI provides very specific starter ideas for us all to get healthy together.

Part VII contains the meal plan and recipes designed specifically for the 10-Day Detox Diet. You will find easy and delicious recipes to follow for each day's meals. There are two plans to choose from: *the Core Plan*, which features simple meals easy enough even for novices in the kitchen, and *the Adventure Plan,* for those who have more time to enjoy cooking and want to experiment with some new flavors and ideas. I'll also give you my "Cooking the Basics" tips with ultrasimple yet delicious vegetables and proteins that you can use as substitutions whenever you are pressed for time.

Online 10-Day Detox Diet Course: Do It Together

Most people don't realize that there is a silver bullet for weight loss — a secret ingredient that, if used correctly, can help you shed pounds and keep them off for good: friends! In fact, when it comes to weight loss, studies show that social threads have a bigger impact than genetics. When people join together to lose weight and get healthy, not only is it more effective, it's also more fun! Losing weight is a team sport. That is why I created an online course for the 10-Day Detox Diet. There you can find Detox Buddies or join a Detox Group and support each other through the process. Need a text at 3:00 p.m. to help encourage you to walk past the cookie jar? We've got you covered! Plus, you'll find videos from me and essential tools to help automate the process: menus, automatic shopping lists, interactive tracking tools, cooking tips and advice, one-click ordering for supplies, journaling tools, automated reminders, and even an app to help you use your Detox on the go. It's everything you need to make your Detox easy to use and to share. Just go to www.10daydetox.com/resources to learn more and sign up.

RESOURCES AND SUPPORT

Everyone needs support and encouragement, to one degree or another, in order to succeed. I encourage you to get the support you need through our online community, through nutrition and life coaching, or through my online 10-Day Detox Diet course, where I will be with you every step of the way with videos, daily webinars, daily e-mails, interactive support, and tips. You will even have the opportunity to join small groups online and detox together. Go to www.10daydetox .com/resources to learn more about the different types of support and communities available to you.

At www.10daydetox.com/resources you will find additional information on where to find the right foods, personal tracking tools, supplements, lab testing, and more. I want you to have all the support you need. Connect, enjoy, and thrive!

A WORD OF CAUTION: YOU MAY WANT TO CONSULT YOUR DOCTOR

I have one strong caution for you before you get started: This program works so well that your blood sugar and blood pressure can drop dramatically in just a day or two. If you are on prescription medication (including blood pressure pills or insulin), you must work with your doctor to carefully monitor your blood pressure and blood sugar, and adjust your doses as necessary. Having your blood sugar or blood pressure run a little high for a week poses almost no danger (if your sugars are under 300 mg/dl and your blood pressure is under 150/100), but rapid drops in blood sugar or blood pressure can be life-threatening. So please be sure to talk with your health care provider before embarking on this journey.

PART I

OUR BIG FAT PROBLEM

1

Why Are We Losing the Weight Loss Battle?

We have a big fat problem.

America is a fat nation, and we are failing to solve our big fat problem. Failing big-time. Almost 70 percent of Americans are overweight. In fact, one in two Americans has what I call diabesity—the spectrum of imbalance ranging from mild insulin resistance to pre-diabetes to full-blown type 2 diabetes. The scariest part is that 90 percent of those suffering from this serious health condition don't even know it (to find out if you have it, take the quiz on the next page).

Being thin today puts you squarely in the minority, and of that thin 30 percent, about one-quarter are what I call skinny fat. That means that while they may not be technically overweight and may even look skinny on the outside, they are fat on the inside, with the metabolic features of a pre-diabetic obese person: low muscle mass, inflammation, high triglycerides, low good cholesterol, high blood sugar, and high blood pressure.

To help you understand why so many people are suffering from similar health problems, I'm going to explain the underlying causes of both the weight-related problems and the chronic diseases that plague us. Then I'm going to show you how you can beat the odds and take back control of your weight and health.

Do I Have Diabesity?

If you answer "yes" to even one of the following questions, you may already have diabesity or are headed in that direction.

Do you have a family history of diabetes, heart disease, or obesity?	
Are you of nonwhite ancestry (African, Asian, Native American, Pacific Islander, Hispanic, Indian, Middle Eastern)?	
Are you overweight (body mass index, or BMI, over 25)? Go to www.10daydetox.com/resources to calculate your BMI based on weight and height.	
Do you have extra belly fat? Is your waist circumference greater than 35 inches for women or greater than 40 inches for men?	
Do you crave sugar and refined carbohydrates?	
Do you have trouble losing weight on a low-fat diet?	
Has your doctor told you that your blood sugar is a little high (greater than 100 mg/dl) or have you actually been diagnosed with insulin resistance, pre-diabetes, or diabetes?	
Do you have high levels of triglycerides (over 100 mg/dl) or low HDL (good) cholesterol (under 50 mg/dl)?	
Do you have heart disease?	
Do you have high blood pressure?	
Are you inactive (less than thirty minutes of exercise four times a week)?	
Do you suffer from infertility, low sex drive, or sexual dysfunction?	
For women: Have you had gestational diabetes or polycystic ovarian syndrome?	

Note: On page 176 of *The Blood Sugar Solution* you can find the comprehensive diabesity quiz, which will tell you if you have basic or advanced diabesity. Or go to www.10daydetox.com/resources and take the online version.

WHY ARE WE FAILING?

Why are nearly 70 percent of Americans and almost 1.5 billion people worldwide—projected to be 2.3 billion by 2015—overweight?

Why do so many of us eat the foods that we know aren't good for us, that cause us to gain weight, that aggravate chronic symptoms, or make us feel sick, bloated, and guilty?

Why would anyone choose to use a substance they know destroys their life?

The answer is simple. Addiction. We are a country—no, make that a world—of food addicts. The industrial food complex has hooked us with a steady stream of hyperprocessed, highly palatable, intensely addictive foods that are sabotaging our brain chemistry, our waistlines, and our health.

THE PROOF IS IN THE MILK SHAKES

The science of food addiction is clearer now than ever before. A powerful study recently published in the *American Journal of Clinical Nutrition* proves that higher-sugar, higher-glycemic foods are addictive in the same way as cocaine and heroin.

Dr. David Ludwig and his colleagues at Harvard proved that foods with more sugar—those that raise blood sugar quickly or have what is called a high glycemic index—trigger a special region in the brain called the *nucleus accumbens* that is known to be ground zero for conventional addictions such as gambling and drug abuse. This is the pleasure center of the brain, which, when activated, makes us feel good and drives us to seek out more of that feeling.

Previous studies have shown how this region of the brain lights up in response to images or when the subject eats sugary, processed, or junk food. But many of these studies used very different foods for comparison. If you compare cheesecake to boiled vegetables, there are many reasons the pleasure center will light up in response to the cheesecake and not to the vegetables. The cheesecake tastes better or it looks better. This is interesting data, but it's not hard proof of addiction.

This new study took on the hard job of proving the biology of sugar addiction. To be certain of their results and to ward off any potential criticism (which the $1-trillion food industry inevitably churns out in response to studies that don't reflect well on its products), the researchers did a randomized, blind crossover study using the most rigorous research design.

They took twelve overweight or obese men between the ages of eighteen and thirty-five and gave each a low-sugar, low-glycemic-index (37 percent) milk shake. Four hours later, they measured the activity of the brain region (*nucleus accumbens*) that controls addiction. They also measured blood sugar and hunger levels.

Then, days later, they had the same subjects back for another round of milk shakes. But this time they switched the milk shakes. They were designed to taste exactly the same, look exactly the same, and *be* exactly the same in every way as the first round of shakes—except in how much and how quickly they spiked blood sugar. In contrast to the first shakes, this second batch of milk shakes was designed to be high in sugar, with a high glycemic index (84 percent).

Not only were the two sets of shakes engineered to deliver precisely the same flavor and texture, they also had exactly the same amount of calories, protein, fat, and carbohydrate. Think of them as trick milk shakes. The participants didn't know which milk shake they were getting, and their mouths couldn't tell the difference, but according to the study results, their brains sure could.

Each participant received a brain scan and blood tests for glucose and insulin after drinking each version of the milk shake. Without exception, they all experienced the same response: The high-sugar, high-glycemic-index milk shake caused a much greater spike in blood sugar and insulin levels, and also yielded reports of increased hunger and cravings four hours after it was consumed.

This part of the study findings was not surprising and had actually been shown in many previous studies. But the breakthrough finding here was this: *When the high-glycemic shake was consumed, the* nucleus accumbens *lit up like a Christmas tree.* By contrast, when the low-glycemic shake was consumed, the *nucleus accumbens* showed no such response. This pattern occurred in every single participant and was statistically highly significant.

This study proved two things. First, that the body responds quite differently to different calories, even if the protein, fat, and carbs (and taste) are exactly the same. And second, **foods that spike blood sugar are biologically addictive.**

So yes, food addiction is very real. Not only is it real; it's the root cause of why so many people are overweight and sick. They are stuck in a vicious cycle of cravings. They eat sugary foods that spike their blood sugar, and their brain's pleasure center lights up. This triggers more cravings, driving them to seek out more and more of the substance that gives them this "high." They are powerless against their brain's hardwired response to seek out pleasure. It's no wonder so many people feel trapped!

ARE YOU ADDICTED TO FOOD?

My friend and colleague Kelly Brownell, PhD, while at Yale's Rudd Center for Food Policy and Obesity, created a scientifically validated food questionnaire to help you determine whether you are a food addict. Here are some clues that you may be addicted to sugar, flour, and processed food. The more intensely or more frequently you experience these feelings and behaviors, the more addicted you are:

- You consume certain foods even if you are not hungry, because of cravings.
- You worry about cutting down on certain foods.
- You feel sluggish or fatigued from overeating.

4. You have spent time dealing with negative feelings after overeating certain foods, instead of spending time in important activities such as time with family, friends, work, or recreation.

5. You have had withdrawal symptoms such as agitation and anxiety when you cut down on certain foods (do not include caffeinated drinks such as coffee, tea, and energy drinks in this).

6. Your behavior with respect to food and eating causes you significant distress.

7. Issues related to food and eating decrease your ability to function effectively (daily routine, job/school, social or family activities, health difficulties), yet you keep eating the way you do despite these negative consequences.

8. You need more and more of the foods you crave to experience any pleasure or to reduce negative emotions.

If you see yourself in these clues, don't worry—you're far from alone. Millions of people in every corner of the world have fallen into the food addiction trap. In this book, you're going to discover once and for all the path that leads you out of biochemical imprisonment and into food freedom.

HOW DID WE GET HERE?

Governments, the United Nations, the Institute of Medicine, and the World Health Organization are all struggling to solve this big fat problem, which accounts for 80 percent of our health care costs and will create a global price tag of $47 trillion over the next twenty years. The National Institutes of Health spends $800 million a year trying to find the "cause" of obesity. Yet despite all this attention, we are still failing.

The causes are multiple, and it's easy to point fingers. Big Food blames lack of exercise and our sedentary lifestyle. Parents blame schools, and schools blame parents. The government won't blame anyone, for fear of losing lobbying and campaign dollars.

The food industry would have us believe obesity is the result of personal choices. Its implication: People are fat because they are lazy and gluttonous, *not* because their biology has been masterfully tricked into craving the toxins that these industries produce. If we all just took more personal responsibility, the industry's paid experts assert, we could solve this problem. There are no good or bad foods, they claim; it's all about moderation. And of course, we should all just exercise a bit more. What they don't explain is that you would have to walk four and a half miles to burn off one twenty-ounce soda. To burn off just one supersize fast-food meal, you'd have to run four miles a day, every day, for a week. Oh, and thanks to the addiction-generating genius of fast-food engineering, once you've eaten that supersize meal, you're going to want another one—soon.

It's true that finger-pointing isn't necessarily going to solve the problem. But I think it's important for us all to understand that the real blame for our weight and health problems lies less with the individuals who've inadvertently become addicted to processed foods than with the food companies that designed food products with highly addictive properties in the first place.

BIG FOOD: THE DRUG PUSHERS

The last few decades have seen the emergence of a whole new breed of "food scientists." Their job is to invent addictive, hyperpalatable processed and junk foods to ensure that their employers (Big Food) get the biggest market share, or what industry insiders call stomach share.

Food scientists focus on creating foods that maximally trigger the "bliss point," that addictive reward pathway in the brain that keeps you coming back for more. They chemically exaggerate certain flavors while suppressing others and alter the chemical structure of fats to enhance the "mouth feel." Their goal: to create a taste sensation so intoxicatingly appealing that no matter how much you eat, you feel you can never get enough.

If the food industry just happened to accidentally create addictive products in an earnest attempt to improve their recipes, we could understand that and expect them to correct their mistake. But these foods happen by design, not by accident.

Big Food spends millions on food science and hires "craving experts" to ensure that its customers will become addicted to deviously developed drugs, all of which are hidden in cleverly disguised delivery vehicles for sugar, fat, and salt. Think heroin lollipops.

You might think I'm paranoid, overstating the case. But in his book *Salt Sugar Fat,* Pulitzer Prize–winning investigative reporter Michael Moss pulls back the veil on Big Food, using meticulous firsthand interviews and research into secret company documents to reveal just how strategically Big Food has altered our food supply to our detriment. Moss points the finger at virtually all the big boys in Big Food and their products, including Kraft, Coca-Cola, Lunchables, Kellogg, Nestlé, Oreos, Cargill, and Capri Sun. (About twelve companies control almost all of the $1-trillion food industry. Frighteningly, they have now also bought up most of the natural and organic food companies.)

Big Food markets the foods just the way Big Tobacco marketed cigarettes, making them "healthier" with come-ons like low tar and nicotine. They might label foods as low-fat or low-salt, but they are hardly healthy, and most still qualify as addictive Frankenfoods. Don't be fooled.

The leading food companies target kids, who can't tell the difference between a TV commercial and a regular show until they are around eight years old. The average two-year-old who is still just learning to talk can cry out in a supermarket for specific brands he or she has seen on television ads. That's scary, because most of the cereals marketed to kids are three-quarters sugar, even the "whole-grain" ones. It is not breakfast. It is dessert! The cereal manufacturers just added "whole grains" when the government recommended we eat more whole grains. Good marketing doesn't make bad food better. It's still a wolf in sheep's clothing. The food is intentionally manipulated to create cravings and addiction. The industry even refers to those of you who buy a lot of their products as heavy users. They know their products are addictive. Now you do, too.

THE PERSONAL RESPONSIBILITY PROPAGANDA

The mantra of the government and food industry is that people should just eat less, choose a "balanced diet," and exercise more. How's that working out for you?

Food addiction is a biochemical problem, not an emotional one. It makes me furious to see patient after patient blame himself or herself for his or her weight problems and diabesity. Yes, we all have choices, and personal empowerment and responsibility are important, but they are not enough if we are trapped in a food coma induced by the toxic influences of sugar and processed foods.

No one chooses to be fat. If you grew up not being able to identify a vegetable because you never ate one, if your school had only deep-fried food or the kind that came out of a box or a can and was stocked with vending machines full of sweetened sports drinks, juices, or sodas, or was ringed by convenience stores where you could buy a sixty-four-ounce Big Gulp on your way home every day, it's no surprise that your habits and taste buds got wired that way.

If nearly every restaurant chain near you serves jumbo portions of sugar and fat and salt, if your workplace lunchroom is a toxic food dump, good luck staying healthy. If, unbeknownst to you, your yogurt contains more sugar than a Coke, and the main ingredient in your barbecue sauce is high-fructose corn syrup, how can the food industry point the finger at you for not taking personal responsibility?

Peer pressure to fit in is strong, and Big Food knows this. Big Food preys on people's desire to be eating and drinking the "in" thing and uses manipulation to get customers hooked. Remember the Coca-Cola ad, "I'd like to buy the world a Coke"? Let's get the whole world hooked! Now North Korea and Cuba are the only countries to which Coke is not distributed. Mission accomplished!

I found a 7UP ad from nearly sixty years ago featuring a baby being fed the soda. The ad proudly boasted that this eleven-month-old was not, "by any means," their youngest customer. The ad with the image of the happy-faced baby went on with gems like these:

> 7-Up is so pure, so wholesome you can even give it to babies and feel good about it.

> By the way, Mom, when it comes to toddlers—if they like to be coaxed to drink their milk, try this: Add 7-Up to their milk in equal parts, pouring the 7-Up gently into the milk. It's a wholesome combination—and it works!

"Wholesome combination"? Who are they kidding?

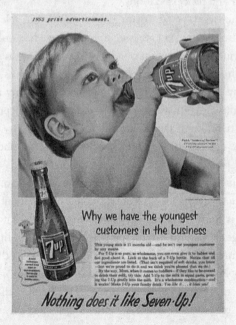

The messages today are subtler, but clearly just as powerful. I remember working in an urgent-care clinic as a resident when a woman came in for an appointment and brought along her seven-month-old baby in a carriage. I saw that the baby was drinking a brown liquid in a baby bottle. I asked the mother what it was and she replied, "Coke." I asked, "Why are you feeding your baby Coke?!" She said, "Because he likes it!"

Of course he did! He was biologically programmed to love sugar and was already an addict at seven months.

When sugar and junk are promoted and accessible in almost every school in America and in the convenience stores that surround them, can we really blame the kids for tripling the childhood obesity rate over the last few decades and for the epidemic of "adult" onset, or type 2, diabetes in seven-year-olds?

If we are feeding our infants, toddlers, and preteens addictive foods and they go on to become obese teenagers and adults hooked on these foods, how can we blame them for lack of "personal responsibility"? There are 600,000 processed food items in our environment, 80 percent of which contain added sugar. Most people have very little opportunity to make (or even understand) healthy choices before the food industry influences their palates and their default food choices for a lifetime.

And yet industry and government still love the personal responsibility story. It allows the food industry to push its addictive products without limit and the government to avoid any politically risky social reform. But when companies profit from getting people to consume more and more of their products—products that are designed to light up our brain's primitive reward center and that have been scientifically proven to cause obesity, heart disease, diabetes, and cancer—we have a problem.

When our government policies and agricultural subsidies have supported the flood of an extra 700 calories per person per day into the food system since 1970 (mostly in the form of high-fructose corn syrup from corn and trans fats), we have a problem.

When government food stamps (the Supplemental Nutrition Assistance Program, or SNAP) pay $4 billion a year for sodas for the poor (29 million servings a day, or 10 billion servings a year) and then the government must pay through Medicaid and Medicare for the obesity, heart disease, diabetes, and cancer caused by soda, we have a problem.

Taylor Swift promotes Diet Coke and footballers promote Pepsi. What if celebrities were featured in billion-dollar ad campaigns aimed at getting kids to try crack cocaine or heroin, all with the promise of a better, happier life? We would all be incensed. But that is essentially what's happening with addictive foods and beverages today in America and, increasingly, around the world.

Nothing less than a comprehensive social and political transformation is needed to hold government and the food and agriculture industries accountable and thus change policy and behavior on a grand scale. We all have to work toward that, and I have outlined many ways to do so in the "Take Back Our Health" section of my book *The Blood Sugar Solution,* and in Part VI of this book.

But in the meantime, we can't wait for food companies to act against their own self-interest, or for the government to regulate the food industry's addictive products and underhanded marketing strategies. We can't wait to free ourselves from the prison of food addiction.

Yes, the food industry has hijacked our taste buds, our brain chemistry, and our biology, but I will show you the keys to breaking free of cravings and life-destroying food addictions. Think of it as a Navy SEAL raid and recovery mission for your health.

Before we get into the active phase of that mission, though, I want you to really understand the science of food addiction. I want to show you precisely how your biology has been influenced. You'll likely be astonished! Please try to read these chapters before diving in. The more aware you are of the biological forces at play—both in terms of how your cravings have been chemically induced and of how easy it is to break free—the more you'll get out of this program. You'll understand not only why this detox works the magic it does, but how to ensure that you never again fall prey to the manipulation of the food industry.

Even more, I'll present to you the overwhelming evidence that *being overweight is not your fault*. Clearly seeing and owning up to your power-lessness in the face of an addiction is the first step of any twelve-step program. We have to start there. Then we can heal.

What I always hated about diets was that I had to think about food every minute of the day. I watched thin people and how they interacted with food, but I was never able to really apply it to my life until now. Now I eat when I'm hungry. I know what's good for me and I eat those foods, and when I'm done, I stop. That's how people without weight issues go about their days. I'm no longer consumed by "Should I eat this, can I eat that?" Now I can think about other things in my life besides food. I love good food, but I'm not consumed by it. That to me is living.

You don't get fat without thinking about how and why. I have had a lot of time to think about what works and what doesn't work, and this program seems different to me because it's freeing. People are slaves to food in so many ways in our society, and it's awful. It's so liberating to see that we really can break free of that control.

—JACKIE WOODS

THE SCIENCE OF FOOD ADDICTION

A little earlier, I mentioned Kelly Brownell, PhD, the former director of the Yale Rudd Center for Food Policy and Obesity. Dr. Brownell recently sent me a copy of his new textbook, *Food and Addiction, A Comprehensive Handbook*. For the first time, it assembles all the latest research into one comprehensive volume on how food addiction is the central driver of obesity and related diseases in our society. I want to share some of Dr. Brownell's most startling findings with you.

Let's break this down into two parts: how food addiction affects our behavior and how it affects our biology.

Food Addiction and Behavior (or Why "You Can't Eat Just One")

> I was a sugar and carbohydrate addict. I couldn't go a day without something sugary. I was like a vampire…I had to have it! I sensed, though, that if I could go a few days without it, I could get past it.
>
> I started the 10-Day Detox and was surprised that I didn't crave sugar. But the way the food plan was designed, I didn't feel hungry or anxious in any way. I was calm, the food was good, and I didn't miss the bad stuff I was eating.
>
> Every day I was on the program I felt more in control…that the food wasn't in control. Before, I used to think, "I know eating this food is bad for me, I know I shouldn't have it, and yet I can't NOT have it." I couldn't stop. I didn't understand that the food literally had physical control over me and that my willpower—even though I had it—wasn't enough. I didn't realize that I was so entrenched in the addiction of the processed foods. They're right with that commercial, you can't have just one! You're sitting there eating it, knowing you shouldn't, yet you cannot stop. I noticed right away that I felt like I was in control over the food, and that was a huge shift.
>
> —JACKIE WOODS

Just as with any other addictive drug, sugar and processed foods cause a temporary high followed by a crash, leading to a vicious cycle of abuse. Food addicts, the research shows, are no different from alcoholics or cocaine addicts. Their lives become increasingly out of control. As their health deteriorates, they gain weight, suffer from arthritis, have trouble getting around or just tying their shoes, and eventually get high blood pressure, diabetes, heart attacks, strokes, and even dementia and depression.

Disordered eating behavior interferes with work or school and family activities. Think about it: It's nearly impossible to focus on your work if you're consumed by thoughts of raiding your colleague's candy dish. It's tough to enjoy a family holiday party with your brain screaming at you to go get another handful of crisps and dip.

Despite wanting to change or stop, those with food addiction cannot resist—even in the face of significant emotional or physical harm to themselves and those they love. They hide their addiction, they worry and obsess about cutting down, all against a backdrop of shame, embarrassment, and denial. They eat a whole sheet cake in the middle of the night in the dark. They say, "It's like someone takes over my body and I can't stop eating. I want to be locked up. I can't keep living this way."

The bottom line is this: Your biology controls your behavior, not the other way around. Yes, if you willfully decide to eat three packages of cookies, your biology will change. But for most of us, most of the time, our biochemistry dictates our behavior.

Our automatic behaviors are controlled by our primitive brain, the neurological machine we have in common with dinosaurs and other reptiles. These automatic behaviors include eating, our fight-or-flight response, and reproduction. This explains why we have so much trouble with food and relationships! According to the primitive brain, survival depends on our avoiding pain (danger) and seeking pleasure (sustenance and safety). When we have a life trauma, this part of our brain is on high alert, making us hypervigilant and protecting us against future threats. This mechanism is so powerful that it can even trigger full-blown post-traumatic stress disorder.

When our brains are bombarded with sugar, a potent pleasure inducer, we become addicted to that pleasure. Willpower and conscious choice are no match for these powerful, ancient drives for survival.

Food Addiction and Biology (aka Stop Blaming Yourself!)

Here's where things get interesting. A 2009 study by Dr. Serge H. Ahmed, *Is Sugar as Addictive as Cocaine?*, published in the journal *Food and Addiction,* proved that **sugar was eight times as addictive as cocaine.** When I first read this, it was hard for me to believe. But this carefully designed study found that when rats were offered intravenous cocaine or sugar (in the form of artificially sweetened water), they always went for the sugar. Even previously cocaine-addicted rats switched to the sweetened water. When higher and higher doses of cocaine were injected intravenously, just below the amount that would give them seizures, they still went for the sweetened water.

Think about it. The rats preferred the equivalent of a Diet Coke to being shot up with intravenous cocaine. Sugary sweetness (in this case created by artificial sweeteners) has a stronger draw than even heroin, which is much more addictive than cocaine. Other studies comparing table sugar and cocaine found the same results, including one done at Connecticut College that showed that rats who were fed Oreo cookies had significantly greater activity in the pleasure center of their brains than those who were injected with cocaine or morphine. And yes, this is an animal study, and rats and humans are different, but the same types of results have been found in human studies.

As I just explained, we are hardwired to seek pleasure and reward. It is a survival mechanism. Anytime we have access to hyperpalatable sweet or fatty foods, we are programmed to eat a lot of them and to store those excess calories as belly fat to sustain us through scarce times that may lie ahead. That's what your body is supposed to do; the problem is that the scarcity we're storing up for never comes. The diabesity epidemic is really just a normal biological response to the inputs from our abnormal environment. What saved us as hunter-gatherers is killing us now.

You're probably wondering why we don't have a built-in control mechanism to tell the brain we have had enough food. We do. Your body's natural brake on hunger is a hormone produced by your fat cells called *leptin*. Unfortunately, in many of us, that natural brake line has been tampered with.

Two bad things happen when your biology is damaged by sugar and processed foods. First, your body becomes *insulin resistant,* so you have to pump out more and more insulin in an attempt to keep your blood sugar normal. Insulin is a powerful fat-storage hormone, one that encourages your body to pack on dangerous belly fat.

Second, you become *leptin resistant*. That means that no matter how much of this fabulous appetite-suppressing hormone your body makes, your brain cannot read the signals. It is "resistant," or numb, to the signals from leptin. But wait...it gets worse.

High levels of insulin produced through all the sugar and fructose consumption (from high-fructose corn syrup and other sugars) block the leptin signals in your brain, so your body thinks it is starving even after a Big Mac, fries, and a large soda. Ever wonder how you can still be hungry right after a big meal? It is the insulin surge and the leptin resistance. This is how sugar and junk food hijack your brain chemistry and your metabolism.

Unfortunately, the story doesn't end there. The fructose (mostly from high-fructose corn syrup) gets directly absorbed from your gut and goes to the liver without passing through the normal controls that glucose has to deal with. Insulin is required to get glucose into the cells, but fructose gets mainlined directly into the liver. This switches on *lipogenesis*, the mechanism that turns sugar directly into fat. Think fatty liver. Think foie gras—not in a goose, but in *you*.

A fatty liver is an inflamed liver. This, in turn, causes even more insulin resistance. Your cells become numb to the effects of insulin, but your body desperately wants to get the sugar into your cells. The body then pumps out more insulin, creating more belly fat and inflammation. This is the cause of most heart attacks and strokes, many cancers, and even dementia. In fact, *insulin resistance is the very cause of aging itself.*

THE PLEASURE CENTER: THE POWER OF SUGAR

Calorie for calorie, sugar is different from other calories that come from protein, fat, or nonstarchy carbs such as greens. As you've seen, it scrambles all your normal appetite controls. So you consume more and more, driving your metabolism to convert it into lethal belly fat. There is no doubt about it: By any definition, sugar is a toxin. Paracelsus, the great medical philosopher, said, *"The dose makes the poison."* We are all overdosed at an average of twenty-two teaspoons of sugar a day per person in America.

Remember the milk shake study? Sugar lights up the pleasure center in the brain and releases dopamine, the "feel-good" chemical. It works on the same parts of the brain as cocaine or heroin, but it is much worse. When researchers provide direct electrical stimulation of the reward centers in the brains of rats, they still can't compete with sugar water. Cocaine lights up only one part of the brain, while sugar lights it up like fireworks on Independence Day!

Brain imaging studies in humans find the same thing. Eating—or even seeing pictures of—junk and processed food lights up the brain like heroin. People say they gain weight just by looking at a donut. They may actually be right, because the body pumps out insulin in response to even the *thought* of something sweet.

When you continue to "use" sugar and processed foods, your dopamine receptors are decreased. That means you need more and more of the addictive substance to generate the same amount of pleasure. This dynamic is called tolerance. It explains why a light or occasional drinker, like me, might feel significant effects from a single alcoholic drink, while a heavy drinker or an alcoholic may need to drink a fifth of vodka just to get a buzz.

When food addicts try to "quit" without proper support, they get withdrawal symptoms lasting up to seven days, including nausea, headaches, shakiness, disorientation, fatigue, cravings, irritability, disturbed sleep, and nightmares. (Don't worry—these symptoms are much less challenging and last for a shorter time when you follow the 10-Day Detox Diet.)

For many, even gastric bypass cannot overcome this addiction. One patient of mine lost 200 pounds (91 kg) through gastric bypass and ate his way back to obesity through a constant stream of M&M's. Too often, gastric bypass fails because it doesn't fix the underlying biology of food addiction.

The Special Case of High-Fructose Corn Syrup

In his book *Fat Chance*, Dr. Robert Lustig calls fructose "the toxin" because it is qualitatively different from other sugars. When fructose occurs naturally, as it does in fruit, with fiber and other nutrients, and when not consumed in excessive quantities, it is fine. But strip fructose out of corn, throw it into a new stew of "free" fructose comprising 55 to 75 percent of the high-fructose corn syrup in sodas (table sugar is 50/50 fructose and glucose), and you have the disaster that is the obesity epidemic.

The high-fructose corn syrup (HFCS) in most of these drinks is worse than regular sugar, despite the propaganda in the multimillion-dollar ad campaign from the Corn Refiners Association rebranding HFCS as natural "corn sugar." The fructose doesn't provide the same feedback control on appetite as regular sugar, making the addiction worse. It fact, it leads to a blocking of the appetite-control hormones, especially *leptin*, the hormone that tells your brain you are full. So you continue to eat and eat, crave and crave, and your body thinks you are starving even though you are drowning in calories. HFCS is the number one source of calories in our diet. As an extra "bonus," high-fructose corn syrup often contains mercury as a by-product of processing.

New research from Dr. Bruce Ames, professor emeritus of biochemistry and molecular biology at the University of California, Berkeley, shows that the free fructose in HFCS causes a leaky gut. Little Lego-like attachments called tight junctions hold the cells of the intestinal lining together. These attachments require energy to stick together. When you eat or drink HFCS, it requires more energy to be absorbed into the body than regular sugar, which depletes the energy supply in the intestinal lining, so those attachments weaken. Food proteins and bacterial toxins then "leak" into your bloodstream through the wall of your intestines, causing your immune system to go into gear and produce system-wide inflammation. The inflammation, in turn, triggers more insulin resistance, weight gain, and diabetes.

So you see, HFCS is *not* just like regular sugar. It has dangerous effects on the body that drive more inflammation, more obesity and diabetes, and more addiction.

LIQUID SUGAR CALORIES (AKA LIQUID DEATH): WHY THEY ARE DIFFERENT FROM REGULAR SUGAR

Remember the rat study? It showed us that sugar-sweetened water (whether sweetened with high-fructose corn syrup or artificial sweeteners) is eight times more addictive than cocaine. Even more than junk food, fast food, or processed carbs such as bread and pasta or chips, sweet drinks have super-addictive properties. While regular old sugary or starchy food will still cause cravings and addiction, the liquid stuff wreaks even more havoc.

It's easy not to notice all those empty calories hidden in sweet drinks. Drinks don't fill you up, which is why, if you include sugar-sweetened and artificially sweetened drinks, you end up eating more total calories in a day. They are easy to consume without thinking about it; we call that passive consumption. They are just drinks, after all. But they add up fast and crowd out real food from your diet. Plus, artificially sweetened drinks jack up your cravings, driving you to eat more food over the course of the day.

Liquid sugar is absorbed very quickly, driving up blood sugar and insulin and mainlining fructose to your liver, setting off a cascade of events that causes weight gain and more cravings. When your insulin spikes and your blood sugar drops, your body sees it as a life-threatening emergency, so you are driven to go looking for your next sugar fix.

It's not just soda we have to worry about, but also sports drinks, sweetened teas and coffees, energy drinks, fruit drinks, and hundreds of other sugary drinks. Ounce per ounce, orange juice has more sugar than cola. If you consume these highly sweetened drinks, your taste buds become adapted to this high-intensity sweetness, and other real, whole food such as vegetables or fruit tastes bland and boring.

Fully 90 percent of kids and 50 percent of the US population drinks soda once a day. One billion cans of Coke are consumed daily around the world. In a review of all the relevant research, scientists found that the number one cause of obesity is sugar-sweetened beverages. One can of soda a day increases a kid's chance of obesity by 60 percent, and in a study of more than 90,000 women, one soda a day increased the risk of diabetes by 82 percent.

One young woman with eight kids from New Zealand had a bad cola habit. It killed her. She drank 2.2 gallons (10 litres) a day, or 2 pounds (450 g) of sugar and 900 milligrams of caffeine. Autopsy reports show she died of a fatty liver and heart damage from the cola. Though the American Beverage Association would have us think otherwise, sugar-sweetened drinks are a major contributor to our big fat problem.

Considering that 15 percent of our calories come from sweetened beverages, cutting them out is an easy way to dramatically improve your health. One patient of mine lost seventy-five pounds (thirty-four kilos) just by becoming aware of and cutting out his liquid sugar calories.

WHY NOT SWITCH TO ARTIFICIAL SWEETENERS?

Diet soda and diet drinks make you fat and cause type 2 diabetes.

Wait...diet soda makes people fat? Really? How does that happen?

If losing weight were all about the calories, then consuming diet drinks would seem like a good idea. That's certainly what Coca-Cola wants us to believe, judging by its ad campaigns highlighting its efforts to fight obesity. (And the other food giants making diet drinks push the same propaganda.) Coke proudly promotes the fact that it has 180 low- or no-calorie drinks and that it has cut sales of sugared drinks in schools by 90 percent.

Is that a good thing? I don't think so. In fact, it may be *worse* to drink diet soda than regular soda. A fourteen-year study of 66,118 women published in the *American Journal of Clinical Nutrition* (and supported by many previous and subsequent studies) discovered some frightening facts that should make us all swear off diet drinks and products:

- Diet sodas raised the risk of diabetes more than sugar-sweetened sodas.
- Women who drank one twelve-ounce diet soda a week had a 33 percent increased risk of type 2 diabetes, and women who drank one twenty-ounce soda a week had a 66 percent increased risk.

- Women who drank diet sodas drank twice as much as those who drank sugar-sweetened sodas because artificial sweeteners are more addictive than regular sugar.
- The average diet soda drinker consumes three diet drinks a day.

Let me lay out a few more of the evils of artificial sweeteners, just in case you're not yet convinced:

- Artificial sweeteners are hundreds to thousands of times sweeter than regular sugar, activating our genetically programmed preference for sweetness more than any other substance.
- Artificial sweeteners trick your metabolism into thinking sugar is on its way. This causes your body to pump out insulin, the fat-storage hormone, which leads to more belly fat.
- Artificial sweeteners confuse and slow down your metabolism, so you burn fewer calories every day. They make you hungrier and cause you to crave even more sugar and starchy carbs, such as bread and pasta.
- In animal studies, the rats that consumed artificial sweeteners ate more food, their metabolic fire or thermogenesis slowed down, and they put on 14 percent more body fat in just two weeks—even if they ate fewer total calories than the rats that ate regular sugar-sweetened food.

The bottom line is that there is no free ride. Diet drinks are not good substitutes for sugar-sweetened drinks. They increase cravings, weight gain, and type 2 diabetes. And they are addictive.

THE WAY OUT

The evidence for biological addiction is overwhelming. You may be saying, "No, not me...I can control my eating. I can handle having some sugar or cookies. It really isn't affecting my life that much."

This is called denial. Food addiction affects more than just a few of the massively obese. It affects nearly all those who are overweight or have struggled to control their eating behavior, cravings, and appetite. The diagnostic criteria for substance abuse in the DSM-V (the psychiatry handbook) match exactly the behavioral characteristics of food addiction, including:

1. Tolerance, the need for increasing amounts of the substance to feel anything (needing more and more to feel good).
2. Withdrawal symptoms from not having the substance.
3. Ingesting larger amounts or over a longer period than intended (bingeing).
4. Persistent desire and unsuccessful attempts to cut down (guilt and shame).
5. Spending a great deal of time to obtain the substance, use the substance, and recover from its effects.
6. Reducing or abandoning significant social, work, or recreational activities.
7. Continuing to use despite awareness of persistent physical or psychological problems that result.

Is there a way out of food addiction? A way to free yourself from the control that processed food and sugar have over your behavior and well-being?

Yes. If we can agree that there is biological addiction, then the only solution is to <u>detox</u> to break the cycle. Try asking a cocaine or heroin addict to "cut down." Forget it. I wish it weren't so, but I am simply the messenger for the science of food addiction. This is why I decided to write this book: to give people powerful tools to painlessly detox from sugar and processed food and reset, reboot, and restore their body to health.

2

Finding Food Freedom

I never thought I could do it...go a week without coffee, without chocolate, without wine, without cheese, etc. But I knew I had to make a
drastic change and needed a jump start. I was very overweight, high
cholesterol, pre-diabetic, and miserable. This has been an amazing gift. I
am not saying that I don't still have thoughts about the above, but they
don't consume me and I feel like I finally have control. Prior to this
detox, I spent every free thought beating myself up for my food choices
and how I looked and felt. Now I am celebrating my accomplishments
(down twelve pounds and in a normal fasting glucose range) and feel
empowered. The biggest gift, though, is that I am finally out of the
"food fog" that I have spent years in. I feel clear, awake, and alert. When
I spend time with my children I feel present and engaged, which is a
blessing for us all. This journey is just beginning and I have a long way to
go and a lot to learn, but I have never been so excited and so over-
whelmingly grateful.

— KELLY ARONSON

It's time to take back control. No more blaming yourself. No more
emotional wrestling or steeling yourself (fruitlessly) with willpower.
You need to use science, not willpower. With this program, you're
going to discover the scientifically proven tools for detoxing your body
and mind and free yourself—once and for all—from the grip of food
addiction.

The key to detoxing is to not just stop all the addictive foods and
substances all at once (which you do need to do), but to immediately

replace them with specific hormone-balancing, brain-healing foods and lifestyle habits. This program detoxes more than just your body: We're going to give you a chance to detox (and reboot) your entire life. We're going to address all the root causes of weight gain, diabetes, and chronic disease, starting with the most powerful tool of all: your mind.

FIXING OUR FAT THINKING

The biggest challenge you're facing here is not your waistline or your weight. It's not your belly. It's your brain. Changing the way you think about food so you get your mind working with your body, not against it, is critical to weight loss and healing.

If you want to lose pounds, you need to first lose the ideas that keep you stuck in an endless cycle of yo-yo dieting. You need to let go of the beliefs and perspectives that sabotage your goal of permanent weight loss and vibrant health. Thinking the way you've always thought and doing things you've always done will only lead to more of the same. You need to be disruptive!

The Blood Sugar Solution 10-Day Detox Diet is meant to be disruptive. Very disruptive. It will go against a lot of what you've been told. That's because the vast majority of conventional nutritionists and doctors have it mostly wrong when it comes to weight loss. Let's face it: If their advice were good and doable, we would all be thin and healthy by now. But as a general rule, it's not. And the mainstream media messages often confuse things even more. So before you get started on this detox, I want to blow up some of the common myths that keep us fat and sick.

MYTH #1: ALL CALORIES ARE CREATED EQUAL

Take a class of sixth graders. Show them a picture of 1,000 calories of broccoli and 1,000 calories of soda. Ask them if they have the same effect on our bodies. Their unanimous response will be "NO!" We all intuitively know that equal caloric amounts of soda and broccoli can't be the same nutritionally. But as Mark Twain said, "The problem with common sense is that it is not too common."

I guess that is why the medical profession, nutritionists, our government, the food industry, and the media are all still actively promoting the outdated, scientifically disproven idea that all calories are created equal. Yes, that well-worn notion—that as long as you burn more calories than you consume, you will lose weight—is simply dead wrong.

Newton's first law of thermodynamics states that the energy of an isolated system is constant. In other words, in a laboratory, or "isolated system," 1,000 calories of broccoli and 1,000 calories of soda are, in fact, the same. I'm not saying Newton was wrong about that. It's true that when burned in a laboratory setting, 1,000 calories of broccoli and 1,000 calories of soda would indeed release the same amount of energy.

But sorry, Mr. Newton; your law of thermodynamics doesn't apply in living, breathing, digesting systems. When you eat food, the "isolated system" part of the equation goes out the window. The food interacts with your biology, a complex adaptive system that instantly transforms every bite.

To illustrate how this works, let's follow 750 calories of soda and 750 calories of broccoli once they enter your body. First, soda: 750 calories is the amount in a Double Gulp from 7-Eleven, which is 100 percent sugar and contains 186 grams, or 46 teaspoons, of sugar. Many people actually do consume this amount of soda. They are considered the "heavy users."

Your gut quickly absorbs the fiber-free sugars in the soda, fructose, and glucose. The glucose spikes your blood sugar, starting a domino effect of high insulin and a cascade of hormonal responses that kicks bad biochemistry into gear. The high insulin increases storage of belly fat, increases inflammation, raises triglycerides and lowers HDL, raises blood pressure, lowers testosterone in men, and contributes to infertility in women.

Your appetite is increased because of insulin's effect on your brain chemistry. The insulin blocks your appetite-control hormone leptin. You become more leptin resistant, so the brain never gets the "I'm full" signal. Instead, it thinks you are starving. Your pleasure-based reward center is triggered, driving you to consume more sugar and fueling your addiction.

The fructose makes things worse. It goes right to your liver, where it starts manufacturing fat, which triggers more insulin resistance and causes chronically elevated blood insulin levels, driving your body to store everything you eat as dangerous belly fat. You also get a fatty liver, which generates more inflammation. Chronic inflammation causes more weight gain and diabesity. Anything that causes inflammation will worsen insulin resistance. Another problem with fructose is that it doesn't send informational feedback to the brain, signaling that a load of calories just hit the body. Nor does it reduce ghrelin, the appetite hormone that is usually reduced when you eat real food.

Now you can see just how easily 750 calories of soda can create biochemical chaos. In addition, the soda contains no fiber, vitamins, minerals, or phytonutrients to help you process the calories you are consuming. These are "empty" calories devoid of any nutritional value. But they are "full" of trouble. Your body doesn't register soda as food, so you eat more all day long. Plus, your taste buds get hijacked, so anything that is not super-sweet doesn't taste very good to you.

Think I'm exaggerating? Cut out all sugar for a week, then have a cup of blueberries. Super-sweet. But eat those same blueberries after bingeing on soda and they will taste bland and boring.

Now let's look at the 750 calories of broccoli. As with the soda, these calories are made up primarily (although not entirely) of carbohydrates— but let's clarify just what that means, because the varying characteristics of carbs will factor significantly into the contrast I'm about to illustrate.

Carbohydrates are plant-based compounds comprised of carbon, hydrogen, and oxygen. They come in many varieties, but they are all technically sugars or starches, which convert to sugar in the body. The important difference is in how they affect your blood sugar. High-fiber, low-sugar carbohydrates such as broccoli are slowly digested and don't lead to blood sugar and insulin spikes, while table sugar and bread are quickly digested carbs that spike your blood sugar. Therein lies the difference. Slow carbs like broccoli heal rather than harm.

Those 750 calories of broccoli make up 21 cups and contain 67 grams of fiber (the average American consumes 10 to 15 grams of fiber a day). Broccoli is 23 percent protein, 9 percent fat, and 68 percent carbohydrate, or 510 calories from carbs. The "sugar" in 21 cups of broccoli is the equivalent of only 1.5 teaspoons; the rest of the carbohydrates are the low-glycemic type found in all nonstarchy vegetables, which are very slowly absorbed.

Still, are the 750 calories in broccoli really the same as the 750 calories in soda? Kindergarten class response: "No way!" So why do we all think that's true, and why has every major governmental and independent organization bought into this nonsense?

Let's take a closer look at just how different these two sets of calories really are.

First, you wouldn't be able to eat twenty-one cups of broccoli, because it wouldn't fit in your stomach. But assuming you could, what would happen? They contain so much fiber that very few of the calories would actually get absorbed. Those that did would get absorbed very slowly. There'd be no blood sugar or insulin spike, no fatty liver, no hormonal chaos. Your stomach would distend (which it doesn't with soda; bloat from carbonation doesn't count!), sending signals to your brain that you were full. There would be no triggering of the addiction reward center in the brain. You'd also get many extra benefits that optimize metabolism, lower cholesterol, reduce inflammation, and boost detoxification. The phytonutrients in broccoli (glucosinolates) boost your liver's ability to detoxify environmental chemicals, and the flavonoid kaempferol is a powerful anti-inflammatory. Broccoli also contains high levels of vitamin C and folate, which protect against cancer and heart disease. The glucosinolates and sulphorophanes in broccoli change the expression of your genes to help balance your sex hormones, reducing breast and other cancers.

What I'm trying to illustrate here (and this is probably the single most important idea in this book) is that **all calories are NOT created equal.** The same number of calories from different types of food can have very different biological effects.

Some calories are addictive, others healing, some fattening, some metabolism-boosting. That's because, as you'll read in "Myth #2" below, food doesn't just contain calories, it contains information. Every bite of food you eat broadcasts a set of coded instructions to your body—instructions that can create either health or disease.

So what will it be, a Double Gulp or a big bunch of broccoli?

Soda and Diabetes

If you still think a calorie is just a calorie, maybe this study will convince you otherwise. In a study of 154 countries that looked at the correlation of calories, sugar, and diabetes, scientists found that adding 150 calories a day to the diet barely raised the risk of diabetes in the population, but if those 150 calories came from soda, the risk of diabetes went up by 700 percent.

MYTH #2: YOU CAN'T FIGHT GENETICS

It's easy to think your biology is a lottery. You got that fat gene, that diabetes gene. Not much you can do about it. Your parents are overweight, your grandparents were overweight, and diabetes runs in your family. Might as well throw in the towel.

The good news is that we have decoded the human genome. Scientists have scoured the genome in the hope of finding the magic key to obesity and diabetes. The bad news is that they didn't find anything terribly helpful to the overweight among us.

There are thirty-two genes associated with obesity in the general population. Unfortunately, they account for only 9 percent of obesity cases. Even if you had all thirty-two obesity genes, you would put on only about twenty-two pounds (ten kilos) of weight. Our genes only change 2 percent every 20,000 years. Since obesity (not just being overweight) has risen from 9 percent to 36 percent since 1960 and is projected to go to 50 percent by 2050 if current trends continue, something other than genetics has to be to blame.

In truth, it's probably lots of things. Over the last 10,000 years, our food supply has changed dramatically, with sugar consumption going from twenty teaspoons a year to twenty-two teaspoons a day. Toxins (which we now know cause obesity and are thus called *obesogens*) have flooded the environment. Our gut flora became toxic because of our high-sugar, high-fat, and low-fiber diet, and this has triggered a huge rise in "micro-obesity"—weight gain due to inflammatory gut bacteria. Sleep debt (Americans sleep two hours less a night than they did a hundred years ago) and obesity-causing viruses have also been implicated. And then there is peer pressure: We imitate the behavior of people in our social network. Research shows we are more likely to be overweight if our friends are overweight than if our parents are overweight. The social threads that connect us may be more important than the genetic ones. There are a hundred reasons, but the least of them are genetics.

Yes, we are programmed to love sugar and fat. We are programmed to store belly fat in response to sugar so that we can survive the winter when food is scarce. Genes do play a role, but they are a minor contributor to the massive obesity and diabetes pandemic we are facing globally. China is a perfect example of the influence of the Western diet in the global marketplace. When I traveled throughout China thirty years ago, I saw one overweight woman, and she was riding a bicycle. Type 2 diabetes was almost unknown. Now China has the most diabetics in the world, and one in five Chinese over sixty has type 2 diabetes. The Pima Indians had no obesity, diabetes, or chronic disease a hundred years ago; now they are the second most obese group in the world (after the Samoans). Eighty percent have type 2 diabetes by the time they are thirty years old.

Perhaps the most important piece of news when it comes to genes and weight is this: **You can put your genes on a diet and program them for weight loss and health.** Yes, you heard that right. You can't swap out the genes you have inherited, but you can literally *reprogram* your genes to help you get slim and healthy.

How? That's easy. Through food.

As I mentioned before (and I will mention it again, because I consider this perhaps the single biggest medical discovery of this century), food contains not just calories or energy to fuel our cells; *food contains information*. It is the control mechanism that regulates almost every chemical reaction in our bodies by communicating instructions to our genes, telling them whether to gain or lose weight, and to turn on the disease-creating or health-promoting genes. This is the groundbreaking science of *nutrigenomics*.

With every bite of food you take, you are sending direct messages to your genes, which control the production of all proteins in your body. And the proteins (hormones, neurotransmitters, and all sorts of chemical messengers) are the very things that control your metabolism, appetite, and health.

When you think about it that way, suddenly choosing the right foods seems like a no-brainer! It all comes down to quality. **Whole, real, and fresh:** Those are the three key words you need to know when it comes to choosing foods to program your genes for weight loss and health. Everything else should be considered "not food."

Think of yourself as a *qualitarian*. Your diet for the upcoming ten days (and hopefully forevermore) will be packed with real, high-quality, whole, fresh foods to put your genes on a diet and make the pounds disappear.

Epigenetics: A Wrinkle in the Gene Story

We know you can't modify your genetic code. But we also know that you can change how your genes function, which ones are activated or silenced by what you eat. New research has found a way to switch genes on and off or affect how they work. This science is called epigenetics.

You have 8 billion letters in your genetic code, or "book of life." Quite a big book! The code won't change, but which letters get "read" does change based on inputs from the outside — starting in your mother's womb. The environment created for you in the womb — what foods, stress, and toxins she was exposed to — will determine how your genes get set for life. This "reading" or bookmarking is how epigenetics determines much of what happens to you during your lifetime. If your mother ate sugar and junk food and was deficient in vitamins and minerals, the messages from the sugar and nutritional deficiencies will get programmed into your genes and increase your risk of obesity and diabetes.

What's worse is that those changes can then get transmitted to your offspring. So what your grandmother ate during her pregnancy, and what toxins she was exposed to, will influence your genes and your grandchildren's genes and risk of disease. But like a cycle of abuse in families, this cycle can be broken.

Switching to real food, optimizing your nutrient status, and lowering your load of environmental toxins can help you reprogram your genes in this lifetime. You can change the bookmarks in your book of life so your body is consistently reading instructions from the slim, healthy chapters — not the fat, sick ones.

MYTH #3: I CAN USE WILLPOWER TO CONTROL MY CRAVINGS

How long can you hold your breath underwater? If I tell you to use your willpower to hold your breath for fifteen minutes and that I will give you a million dollars if you do, there is still no way you can do this. We are programmed for certain needs: air, water, food, sleep, and sex. These things are essential to our survival. If you are addicted to sugar and I tell you to resist giving in to your cravings by using willpower, I might as well tell you to hold your breath for fifteen minutes. It won't work.

No one *wants* to be overweight or suffer the emotional or physical consequences of diabetes or obesity. But willpower simply isn't enough to overcome the cravings for crisps, cookies, soda, and more. We're up against powerful biochemical mechanisms created by food addiction. Willpower is useless when industrial junk food and sugar are in charge of your brain chemistry.

The very good news is that breaking these addictions is easier than you might think—if you know what to do. And it doesn't take weeks or months. Simply following the exact instructions in the 10-Day Detox Diet will quickly reset your brain chemistry and give you back control over your eating behavior. You don't have to struggle to let go of your cravings; your cravings will naturally let go of you.

Your body is an extraordinary instrument—a thing of wonder that when tuned to the right frequency plays the most beautiful songs of well-being, balance, health, and energy. The trick is to tune up your biology, tune up your hormones, and tune up your metabolism so everything plays in harmony. When that happens (and on this program, it will), you'll find that your cravings disappear very quickly—generally within a day or two. It does take a little leap of faith, but please take that leap; your body knows what to do!

> This has been one of the best experiences of my life. I have confidence that I can get my weight down to normal and live to be a healthy old girl. No suffering. To break my addictions with no pain has been truly remarkable. I didn't know I could do it without hunger...I cannot thank you enough.
>
> —DIANA STEUF

MYTH #4: YOU CAN BE HEALTHY
IF YOU ARE OVERWEIGHT

A research finding got big headlines recently. "New Study Finds That Overweight People Have Lower Death Rates Than Thin People." Nonsense. This makes for sensational headlines, but looking at the real facts of this and other studies helps to clarify that being overweight negatively impacts your health and longevity in a number of ways.

The study analyzed 100 other studies encompassing 2.88 million people with over 270,000 deaths. Those who were overweight based on a BMI (body mass index) of 25 to 30 seemed to have a lower risk of death than those who were skinnier, with a body mass index of 18.5 to 25. However, those who were obese, with a BMI of *more* than 30, had a much higher risk of death. Is the take-home message that you should gain more weight to live longer? Hardly.

There are many problems with the study. It included very skinny people in the "normal weight" group, people who are often quite sick, like my sister, who recently died of cancer and was rail thin at her death. Chronically ill people, especially those with cancer, die very thin. In fact, the lowest risk of death was in the group with a BMI of 22 to 25.

Other factors also confuse this study. Body mass index doesn't account for how much of your weight is from body fat or muscle mass. Shaquille O'Neal, one of the greatest basketball players in history, has a BMI of 35 (which is considered morbidly obese), but he is muscular, not fat. You can also be what I call a skinny-fat person, with a low body mass index but very little muscle; even though you are of normal weight, you are fat on the inside. If you have skinny arms and legs and a big belly, you may be of normal weight but still have a high risk of death.

The only way to correlate weight with mortality is to look at muscle and fat composition, as well as disease markers such as high blood pressure, cholesterol, blood sugar, insulin, inflammation, and other markers that show you how sick you are independent of weight.

This was also a global study, and it is well known that Asians and East Indians can have diabetes at much lower body weights. So while interesting, this study doesn't prove anything significant, and it certainly doesn't suggest that you can carry excess weight without also carrying increased risks of chronic disease and premature death.

There is also some research that says if you are overweight but fit, your risk of disease is lower. Certainly fitness at any weight reduces the risk of disease and death, but to promote the benefits of being fat and fit only suits the food industry. In fact, the Center for Consumer Freedom, a food and tobacco industry front group, published a white paper on the "obesity hoax." The liberal media and the government, they say, are perpetrating a big hoax on Americans. We are not fat, they insist, and diabetes is not on the rise. Oh, please! If you believe that, just take a walk through your local mall.

The Center for Consumer Freedom is funded by Coca-Cola, Monsanto, Philip Morris Kraft (which changed its name to Altria to escape negative cigarette- and junk-food-related brand perceptions), and other food industry giants—though on their website they hide the sponsors; maybe they fear attack by food activists, those militant, vegetable-eating terrorists. Oh my!

These are the same companies that espouse the wonders of pesticides and oppose bans on smoking in public places. The group defines its mission as fighting against "a growing cabal of food cops, health care enforcers, militant activists, meddling bureaucrats, and violent radicals who think they know what's best for you, [who] are pushing against our basic freedoms."

"Don't believe your eyes," implies the Center for Consumer Freedom. The Center maintains that contrary to all the observable data, we are *not* a fat nation. It's just all those food fascists confusing us, including food and nutrition experts from Yale, Harvard, and similar second-rate institutions. What's scariest is that this industry front group has more than 100,000 Facebook likes.

What's the group's advice? "Instead of focusing solely on food, focus on physical activity." Really? Remember, you have to run for four miles every single day for one week to burn off just one supersize fast-food meal. But of course *that* doesn't show up anywhere in the Center's report.

My counsel is this: Don't believe the sensational headline hype, and don't take health advice from industry front groups. Do pay attention to the toll that excess weight is taking on your vitality. Because what a huge body of scientific literature really shows us is that obesity comes with a whole set of metabolic changes and imbalances that create a smoldering fire of pre-disease that often leads to full-blown disease.

There are a very few people who can be overweight and metabolically healthy, but they are anomalies. Most have dangerous inflamed belly fat, abnormal small cholesterol particles (the ones that cause heart attacks), high blood pressure, and high levels of insulin, causing both insulin and leptin resistance. Their sex hormones are messed up, causing sexual dysfunction in men, and infertility, hair loss on the head, facial hair, abnormal menstrual cycles, and acne in women. Their blood is inflamed and more likely to clot and cause heart attacks and strokes. Their risks of breast, colon, prostate, pancreatic, liver, and kidney cancer are increased. Their excess weight overloads their joints, causing arthritis and mobility issues. And many have depression, memory problems, and "pre-dementia," all caused by hormones and biochemistry disrupted by belly fat. In fact, Alzheimer's is now being called type 3 diabetes.

So no, it is not wise to kick back and think you are fine if you are a bit overweight. Get your biomarkers tested and really find out. The basic tests you need are listed on page 73. Go to www.10daydetox.com/resources to learn more about these tests, which will help determine whether your weight is putting your health in jeopardy.

MYTH #5: EXERCISE IS THE KEY TO WEIGHT LOSS

If you think you can exercise your way to weight loss, I am sorry to say you are in for a big disappointment. Do you treat yourself to a post-workout sugar-laden smoothie, muffin, or other "healthy" snack? Suck back some Gatorade to quench your thirst after your thirty minutes on the treadmill? While some after-sports snacks can help enhance repair and recovery, for most of us, unless you are an endurance athlete or run around like Kobe Bryant for forty-eight minutes on the basketball court at full speed, they are causing more harm than good. In fact, using exercise to lose weight without changing your diet is asking for failure. You can change your diet and lose weight, but if you exercise and keep your diet the same, you may gain some muscle, improve endurance, and be healthier overall, but you won't shed many pounds.

Remember, if you consume one twenty-ounce soda, you have to walk four and a half miles to burn it off. If you consume one supersize fast-food meal, you have to run four miles a day for one whole week to burn it off. If you eat that every day, you have to run a marathon every single day to burn it off.

The simple fact is that you cannot exercise your way out of a bad diet.

Having said that, I don't want you to get the impression I don't think exercise is important. It is an essential component of the Blood Sugar Solution 10-Day Detox Diet. Exercise is critical, but not for the reasons you think. Here's how exercise helps and why we need it:

- It makes your cells and muscles more sensitive to insulin so you don't need as much. Less insulin = less belly fat.
- It reduces the stress hormone cortisol. Too much cortisol and you become insulin resistant and store belly fat. Too much cortisol also makes you crave sugar and carbs and seek comfort food.
- If you do interval training (going fast and then slow, as with the wind sprints you did in high school), you can speed up your metabolism and burn more calories all day long, even while you sleep.
- Strength training builds muscle, and muscle burns seven times as many calories as fat. Even if you are skinny, strength training is key because it prevents "skinny fat" syndrome.
- Exercise improves memory, learning, and concentration.

- Vigorous exercise is a better antidepressant than Prozac.
- Exercise protects your heart and reduces your risk of heart attack and stroke.
- Exercise reduces inflammation (the cause of almost every disease of aging).
- Exercise boosts detoxification of environmental chemicals.
- Exercise balances hormones and reduces breast and other common cancers.
- Exercise improves sexual function.

Speaking of sex, there is one more little myth I need to blow up for you. Somewhere we all got the idea that sex was good exercise and that a bout of sexual activity burns 100 to 300 calories for each participant. That reminds me of a patient I saw when I was a resident. I asked her if she was sexually active. She said, "No, I usually just lie there." But even if you don't just lie there, a vigorous lovemaking episode usually lasts about six minutes (the average in America) and burns about twenty-one calories. If you just sat and watched TV, you would burn fourteen calories in the same time. So find other ways to exercise, or study tantric sex and strive to make love for an hour or more.

Just know that even then, you probably still can't "love" your way to weight loss. You'll have to get out of bed and start moving—and you'll still need to change the way you eat.

MYTH #6: YOU HAVE TO BE "READY" TO SUCCEED AT WEIGHT LOSS

A recent analysis of weight loss research by the *New England Journal of Medicine*, entitled *Myths, Presumptions and Facts about Obesity*, attempts to bust some of the myths about weight loss and explains why many common strategies fail. One of the wrongheaded ideas it addresses that has pervaded the weight loss world is this idea that you need to be "ready to change" in order to succeed.

While there is some truth to that (certainly, if you refuse to even *try* something new, you're not going to get very far), based on my experience in treating tens of thousands of patients over the decades, I see it a little differently.

What I've seen over and over again is that once people embark on a program that actually *works*, they get immediate positive feedback that makes

I don't have to look far to see what's in the history of my family: COPD (emphysema) and congestive heart failure, which is what my dad died of. My mom has congestive heart failure now, too. My sister was diagnosed with type 2 diabetes and is on insulin. I have too many kids and grandkids to live for, and I realize that the time to get healthy is NOW. It's one thing to realize this, but it's another thing to act on it. It's time to start seeing my health as a priority and acting on it.

—BILL COTEE

them inclined to continue. Even if they didn't start out feeling particularly ready or committed to make lasting changes, those results inspire them to get ready—fast.

So even if you don't feel inspired or excited or motivated to start taking care of yourself, do it anyway. You are just as likely to succeed as someone who is highly motivated. Simply give this program a few days and you'll start seeing results that will not only increase your readiness to change, but will also deliver the change you've been hoping for.

MYTH #7: IF YOU MAKE SMALL CHANGES IN YOUR LIFESTYLE, YOU WILL LOSE WEIGHT

This is another myth tackled in the *New England Journal of Medicine* analysis. We have been taught to make small changes in our diet and lifestyle to create the most success. If the small change is cutting out the daily sixty-four-ounce Double Gulp, then yes, that will make a difference. But most need to make big changes to see big results.

For example, most of us have learned that if we just cut our intake by 100 calories a day, or increase our exercise a little bit over the long haul, we will lose weight. We're continually told that it's all about the calories in, calories out. But as you saw earlier in the broccoli vs. soda comparison, biology and metabolism are far more complex than that.

Just going with the math, if you burned an extra 100 calories a day (walking one mile) or consumed 100 calories less per day over thirty-five days, you would lose a pound (3,500 calories = 1 pound/450 g). So, in theory, over five years you would lose fifty pounds or 23 kilos. Yet studies show that in reality you're more likely to lose only ten pounds (4.5 kg) in five years, not fifty. Why? Because of changes in your metabolism and caloric needs that occur as you lose weight. You'll need to consume even fewer calories, or burn even more of them, just to keep losing at the same rate. For most people, this pace of progress is totally demotivating, which is why they generally abandon their small-scale diet and exercise attempts early on.

Bottom line: Big changes are needed to create big weight loss. That is why the Blood Sugar Solution 10-Day Detox Diet creates big, high-impact changes right from the start. The program will jump-start the process and unhook you from the cycle of failure and frustration that comes from making small changes that lead to small or no results.

MYTH #8: DON'T LOSE WEIGHT TOO FAST OR YOU WILL REBOUND AND GAIN IT ALL BACK

The most difficult aspect of being morbidly obese for me has been adhering religiously to the latest "best" diet, losing five to ten pounds and then stalling for weeks. It is eating under 1,000 calories a day, walking daily in the hot, humid Southern summer until I cannot walk another step, and losing maybe .25 pound per week. Having my health care provider look at me skeptically as I present my carefully detailed dietary intake log, and being asked, "Now what have you really been eating?"

In the past, to lose weight I have had to reduce my nutritional intake until I was dizzy most of the time and my hair began falling out. Even then I would plateau and the scale wouldn't budge. And I would think, "It is just not worth it." It was hard for me to try yet again, but I trust Dr. Hyman and his functional approach to health promotion. So I joined the trial program, afraid to hope in case this was one more unsuccessful attempt.

But after ten days I lost 14.2 pounds and 6.5 inches. My fasting glucose was down ten points, in the low eighties. It had taken me four years to lose forty pounds, and now all of a sudden 14.2! In ten days!! I have adopted a new approach to nutrition, and am so very grateful.

— JANITH KATHLENE WILLIAMS

This is another wrongheaded idea that the *New England Journal of Medicine*'s report burst open. We have (incorrectly) learned that rapid weight loss always backfires. We have been taught that if you go for the quick fix, you won't lose as much in the long run as if you take the slow, gradual approach. But that is not necessarily true. Studies show that if you drop weight quickly, you end up with more weight loss in the end. When I give my patients a big jump start with weight loss, they do better and lose more weight over the long run. They learn how to own their bodies and feel empowered. The studies back up the results I see with my patients.

The key is to use a healthy, sustainable strategy for weight loss that balances your hormones and brain chemistry and doesn't put you in a starvation response. The truth is that you can and should kick-start significant weight loss with dramatic (but healthy) shifts in your diet. That is why the Blood Sugar Solution 10-Day Detox Diet is so effective. It gives you fast, safe, powerful results that set you up for long-term, sustained weight loss when supported by the transition programs you'll find in Part V of this book or the program outlined in *The Blood Sugar Solution*.

3

The Solution: The 10-Day Detox Diet

Now that you understand the biology of food addiction and the means by which sugar takes hold of your taste buds, your hormones, your brain chemistry, and your waistline, and now that you know what controls hunger and fat storage, you can use that knowledge to achieve a healthy weight and metabolism not by willpower but by detoxification. It's time for rehab!

Once you take back control of your biochemistry and body, you can be more flexible, but at the beginning you have to think about this as you would any other addiction. You must unhook from the biology that drives your behavior.

It takes dramatic change to reset your biology when it is in a state of chaos. You know how when your computer freezes, you need to reboot the whole system? You can't just shut down one program and hope it will right itself. Well, you need to do something similar to regain control of your health.

Remember, biochemistry drives your behavior, not willpower. So you'll have to use some biochemical science to reset your hormones and neurotransmitters—and by extension, to effortlessly end your cravings, lose weight, and reverse disease. That science is the foundation of the Blood Sugar Solution 10-Day Detox Diet.

Here's what the detox will do for you:

1. **Shut down the insulin surges**—and thereby arrest belly fat storage and cravings.

2. **Improve your cells' sensitivity to insulin** so you need less to balance your blood sugar, resulting in weight loss and health.
3. **Reduce cortisol**—the stress hormone that increases cravings for sugar, promotes belly fat storage, and shrinks your brain.
4. **Lower ghrelin**, the hunger hormone.
5. **Improve leptin sensitivity** in the brain, allowing your natural appetite-regulating system to begin to work again.
6. **Increase the brake on appetite called PYY** (peptide YY), the intestinal hormone that makes you feel full after a meal.
7. **Increase dopamine naturally** and reset your brain's reward pathways so you can feel pleasure from eating real food.
8. **Reset your taste buds** so real food tastes good again.
9. **Reduce inflammation** (the problem at the root of almost all weight gain and chronic disease) by eliminating common food sensitivities, processed foods, and sugar and by including anti-inflammatory foods.
10. **Boost detoxification** by eliminating toxins from your diet and life and enhancing your body's ability to get rid of stored toxins that make you fat.

Each of these important biological changes occurs automatically during the Blood Sugar Solution 10-Day Detox Diet. They happen as you detox from sugar and processed food...as you shift your eating patterns...as you flood your body with real, whole, fresh, anti-inflammatory foods...as you learn the simple, fundamental skills to help your body heal.

Keep in mind, though, that this program is designed not just for easy and rapid weight loss, but also to prepare you for long-term weight management and health improvement. So during each of the ten days, you will also focus on one aspect of whole-system healing. I will teach you how to:

1. **Satisfy** to cut your cravings for sugar and processed food.
2. **Detox** from all addictive substances and support your body's detoxification system.

3. **Empty** and clean out your digestive system to help your body eliminate toxins.
4. **Move** your body so you improve your metabolism to create optimal health.
5. **Listen** to the changes happening in your body and become aware of the natural shifts toward health and wellness.
6. **Think** and examine the thoughts, beliefs, and attitudes that get in the way of weight loss, and create new thought patterns for health and well-being.
7. **Nurture** yourself and calm your nervous system through simple techniques of breathing and relaxation.
8. **Design** your life through focused planning and attention and change your environment to create the automatic conditions for health.
9. **Notice** and track the changes happening in your body, including your food intake, movement, sleep patterns, and numbers (weight, waist size, blood pressure, blood sugar, lab tests, and medical symptoms).
10. **Connect** with others to get support to sustain and enhance the changes you have made, and to make changes in your community that can help us all heal.

As you progress through this learning experience, you will be simultaneously removing toxins, sugars, processed foods, and chemicals (like artificial sweeteners, preservatives, and MSG), plus foods (like gluten and dairy) that commonly cause allergies and sensitivities. You'll be removing a lot of inflammatory, addictive, health-robbing things from your diet and your life. But what you'll be adding is just as important, if not more so.

The food plan will introduce healing, anti-inflammatory, insulin-balancing, appetite-regulating, and detoxifying foods to your diet. You'll be enjoying foods rich in phytochemicals—powerful, natural compounds that remove weight-producing toxins, including pesticides, heavy metals, and other chemicals known as *obesogens*. You'll also be indulging in some delightful stress-relieving, self-care activities. This program is not about deprivation, but about abundance. It is about new choices and a new experience of health.

QUICK START, LONG-TERM FIX

You might wonder, "How is ten days enough to make a difference? Can I really accomplish anything in ten days that will make a lasting impact?" My answer is yes.

We have learned that if you have diabetes, you can reverse it in a few weeks with a gastric bypass, even if you are still morbidly obese. Why? Because when you rapidly shift your way of eating, you shift your hormones, brain chemistry, and biology very quickly.

Think of the Blood Sugar Solution 10-Day Detox Diet as a gastric bypass without the pain of surgery, vomiting, malnutrition, or weight regain. Research has shown that dramatic changes in diet, *without* gastric bypass, can very quickly normalize blood sugar in type 2 diabetics, getting them off medication in as little as a week. After twelve weeks, their liver, pancreas, and metabolism all return to normal. Your body is capable of amazing healing if you give it the chance.

But as I said, you don't have to believe me. You just have to try it. You can do anything for ten days. The proof will be in the results.

Some may think this program extreme, or dismiss it by saying that if you eliminate any group of foods (like sugar or gluten or dairy), you will lose weight because you reduce overall calories. But this is not a calorie-restricted program, although it is possible that your net calories will naturally go down as the result of eating real food. That's because real, whole foods are nutrient-rich and calorie-poor, whereas processed foods tend to be calorie-rich and nutrient-poor. As I explained in Myth #1, though, this really isn't about calories. If you eat only real, whole, nutrient-dense foods (and stop obsessing about counting calories), you will win every time.

In just a few days you can literally reprogram your biology with the right foods, eaten at the right time with a few other simple lifestyle changes that can allow you to detox painlessly and experience how freeing it is to escape food addiction without struggle. There might be a moment of doubt, or even terror at the thought of giving up your Coke or Diet Coke, or your daily bread or cookies. You might wonder, "If I take away the things that make me feel good (however temporarily), what will I replace them with?"

What I'm offering you in exchange is a radical promise. It's the promise that you will emerge after the first few days of this program feeling light, happy, energetic, and alive again—released from the grip of food addiction and in possession of a vitality you probably haven't experienced in years. The joy you feel from being free of cravings and struggles with food will quickly replace any quick-hit high you get from sugar and junk. All you have to do is take that first step.

If you are looking to get into a special dress or suit for a big event, or to get ready for beach season, or just to do a quick reset on your overall health, it's fine to use those goals as motivators. You will see fast results to get you to those goals. But I want you to understand that the impact of this program is far greater than the achievement of any short-term aspiration. Once you have used the program to reset your biology, you'll see that it is really the beginning of an entirely new way of eating and living—one that will lead to optimal weight and long-term health and vitality.

In the next chapter, you'll discover the potent combination of foods and lifestyle practices that make up the 10-Day Detox. You'll learn everything you need to know, get, and do to radically change your body—and your life—from the inside out.

PART II

ABOUT THE PROGRAM

4

How the Program Works

Now that you know the science of *why* you're doing this program, let's jump in and get to the what, when, who, and how of the Blood Sugar Solution 10-Day Detox Diet.

WHAT YOU'LL DO

> I have had such a hard time over the years gaining any control over my weight, no matter what I have tried. Low-fat, no-fat, low-carb, and on and on and on to no avail. I am so appreciative of this program and thank Dr. Hyman for his dedication to educating us on how to get back our lives in only ten days! It's so easy to love this program, because it's so doable. My weight has dropped about eight pounds, I've lost almost two inches from my waist and one inch from my hips, and my mind has come out of its stupor.
>
> — WENDY FREEMAN

There are three phases of this program, and all are key to your success:

Phase 1, the Prep Phase, is detailed in Part III of this book. There you'll find everything you need to get started and set yourself up for optimal success, beginning with your pantry and ending with your mind-set. Ideally, set aside two days for this phase before you begin the program, to physically and psychologically set the detox process in motion. During those two days, you'll gather all the food and supplies you need. (Those of you who want to order your supplements through my website www.10daydetox.com/resources may want to do that a week before beginning the program, to make sure you have them on hand before you begin.) I'll provide you with a clear checklist with everything you need to get and do during the Prep Phase.

Phase 2, the 10-Day Detox, is outlined for you in Part IV of this book. There you'll find step-by-step directions on what to eat and when during each day of your detox. I'll also give you everything you need to know to do the essential daily practices, including exercise, the UltraDetox Bath, journaling, and daily relaxation exercises (all of which are critical for healing!). Each of the ten days has a specific focus to help you remove the most common obstacles to weight loss success and provide the tool kit to get and stay healthy.

Phase 3, the Transition Phase, is featured in Part V. The Transition Phase gives you a road map for what to do after your 10-Day Detox, and how to transition to a long-term health and weight loss strategy based on my book *The Blood Sugar Solution*. I know you'll want to continue feeling as great as you do immediately after the ten days!

WHAT YOU'LL EAT

This program isn't about deprivation. It's not about eating bland, boring food. That's why the meal plan is filled with flavorful, easy-to-make recipes. Cooking gets a bad rap: It takes too much time…it's inconvenient… it's too difficult, or you don't know how to cook. But the fact is, Americans spend more time watching cooking shows on television than actually cooking!

> I gotta tell you, Dr. Hyman: You should rename that book of yours *A Detox Fit for Foodies*. Your chef is off the hook! I'm a foodie and a pretty good cook and the flavor of these meals is excellent. I'm loving my detox!
>
> — DIERDRE O'CONNOR

We are raising a generation of Americans who don't know their way around the kitchen, where 50 percent of meals are eaten outside the home, and ones eaten at home are usually reheated, factory-made science projects that resemble food but aren't. And as you now know, this convenience is killing us.

You don't have to become a master chef or spend all your time in the kitchen to eat healthfully, but you do need to learn some basic cooking skills. The truth is that if you can read, you can cook. Simply follow recipes step by step and you will usually end up with a great meal.

This is partly how I learned to cook. By simply following recipes for various kinds of dishes, you get a sense of what goes with what, how to use ingredients, and how to naturally flavor and spice foods. These days, I almost never need a cookbook because I've internalized all those principles and feel confident experimenting on my own. I want to help you achieve the same level of kitchen confidence.

Start by deciding to make cooking meals fun. Get family members on board and shop and cook together. Make a point of learning new skills and trying recipes together. Take time to enjoy and celebrate the food you've prepared by hand—as opposed to inhaling something straight from its packaging as you pull out of the fast-food drive-through lane.

Your health depends on cooking, and our national survival depends on health. My friend Pilar Gerasimo (the founding editor of *Experience Life* magazine) says that in a world as health-challenged as ours, "being healthy is a revolutionary act." In part, she explains, this is because it requires all kinds of unconventional choices, a huge amount of conscious determination, and a willingness to learn new skills and strategies. I agree, and for all the same reasons, I also believe that cooking has become a revolutionary act. It's something we must all learn—or relearn—in order to reclaim responsibility for our own well-being and the well-being of future generations.

Michael Pollan, in his book *Cooked*, concurs. He says, "The decline of everyday home cooking doesn't only damage the health of our bodies and our land but also our families, our communities and our sense of how our eating connects us to the world."

He tells us that the effects of not cooking are profound. We have outsourced our cooking to the food industry. When we rely on processed products for our sustenance, we become "consumers" instead of producers of food. We become dependent on corporations and reliant on toxic combinations of salt, sugar, and fat, chemicals that destroy our health, families, and communities. By contrast, getting our hands messy with real food reconnects us to the essential elements that make us human.

Cooking is a uniquely human activity. In fact, taking back our kitchens and embracing the act of cooking real food is probably the single most important thing that any one person can do to create a healthy, sustainable food system. It is also a magical alchemy that transforms individual ingredients into ambrosia and pleasure.

You can choose from two recipe plans during the 10-Day Detox: the *Core Plan* and the *Adventure Plan*. The goal of the Core Plan is to provide quick, simple, and tasty metabolism-boosting meals. The recipes in the Core Plan give you an easy way to succeed in the kitchen and will help convince you that eating well doesn't have to be difficult or complicated. They will also show you that homemade food can delight not just your body, but also your mind and senses, leaving you energized and inspired.

Those of you who have more time to enjoy cooking can opt for the Adventure Plan. These recipes use a wider array of ingredients and allow you to take your exploration of flavors and combinations to a new level. Follow the Adventure Plan for more fun, extra weight loss, and extra health!

Feel free to mix and match between the two plans, as long as you stay within the menu plans listed for each individual day. In other words, if you want to do the Core Plan lunch and the Adventure Plan dinner from Day 3, that's perfectly okay; just don't mix and match the lunches and dinners from different days at random. The daily menus

> When I say I feel like I've gotten my life back, it's because I have a renewed sense of purpose. I am finally succeeding, not getting into a funk because I've failed once again at a weight loss program. I've enjoyed myself this week because I'm surprised at how good healthy food can be…and I'm hopeful that I won't have to live on baked chicken and carrots for the rest of my life! I've reconnected to my love of cooking as I've measured, chopped, minced, and experienced spices and flavors I have never tried before.
>
> — REGINA HURST

are carefully calibrated to make sure you get the right daily dose of nutrients—at the right times of day—to keep you satiated.

Lastly, if you are really pressed for time or don't like either the Core Plan or Adventure Plan recipes for that day (though I encourage you to have an open mind and try them), you always have the option to prepare instead a meal consisting of a basic protein and a nonstarchy vegetable. In Chapter 20, you will find "Cooking the Basics," which gives you super-simple methods for preparing these easy proteins and vegetables.

WHO YOU'LL HAVE ON YOUR SIDE

> The support of the 10-Day Detox online community group was invaluable. Not just for asking cooking questions…to hear everyone's thoughts and feelings was just so precious. If I had a good day, I could share that. And if I didn't, I could share that, too, and get encouragement and support. It was so inspiring when groups of us had similar hurdles to deal with.
>
> — LARRAINE FELDMAN

Knowing what to do is not difficult for most of us. A little knowledge, information, teaching, and instruction and we should all be on our way to health, happiness, fabulous well-being, and our ideal weight. Yet somehow it doesn't work like that.

Despite our best intentions, despite knowing what to eat, and that we should exercise, sleep enough, and de-stress, most of us stumble along in old habits and patterns that keep us from being fully alive and healthy. There may be many deep psychological reasons for this. And after years of psychotherapy, and even abundant use of psychiatric medicine (now second only to cholesterol medication as the most frequently prescribed class of drugs), most of us still find changing our behavior the most difficult thing to do. But I have discovered a little secret that makes change easy and makes it stick.

For years I studied the intricate nature of our human biology, how to turn the dials on all our biological systems to reverse disease and create abundant good health, investigated the finer points of biochemistry and genetics, and yet none of it mattered if my patients couldn't alter their behavior. Some of my patients, of course, had powerful internal motivation, but most needed support. I realized that we are social animals. Those around us, it seems—our families, our friends, our neighborhoods, our schoolmates, our communities, and our workplaces—determine our behavior. As I explained in Part I, the social threads that connect us might in the end be more important than genetics.

After this essential insight about how we change our behavior, I met pastor Rick Warren of Saddleback Church, in Orange County, California, and suggested that we create a healthy living program and deliver it through the thousands of small groups that already existed in his church. These small groups had been formed to help the people within his congregation support and encourage each other, so why not leverage them for physical as well as spiritual renewal and development?

Rick and I both believed that individuals tend to grow and learn better together, and that through sharing, collaboration, and mutual encouragement, they could more effectively express their best selves. So together with Dr. Mehmet Oz and Dr. Daniel Amen, we launched the Daniel Plan on January 15, 2011. It was named after Daniel from the

Bible, who resisted the king's temptation of rich food and ate vegetables and water and was healthier for it.

Initially, we considered the Daniel Plan a social experiment to learn whether community support could be more effective than medication or conventional medical care in treating and reversing disease and creating health. But the results surpassed our wildest expectations.

In the first week, 15,000 people signed up. During the first year, they lost an estimated 250,000 pounds /113,000 kg—the equivalent of ten tractor-trailer trucks loaded with soda. Those results impressed all of us. But here's what we found really interesting: The research indicated that *those who did the plan together lost twice as much weight as those who did it alone.*

The group support was the lever that moved mountains—mountains of donuts, ribs, soda, and more! Beyond the incredible weight reductions, we also saw significant reductions in the participants' doctor visits, hospitalizations, and need for medications.

In a survey taken ten months after the launch of the program, participants reported the following:

- 53 percent had increased energy.
- 34 percent reported better sleep.
- 27 percent saw an improvement in blood work.
- 20 percent saw an improvement in blood pressure.
- 11 percent cut down on their medications.
- 31 percent reported improvement in mood.

We didn't treat disease. We didn't create a weight loss program. We taught people self-care, and combining that with caring for each other, they created a miracle—something that health care or health care reform has not been able to achieve. People helped each other create health. We realized that the group was the medicine, that the community was the cure, and that most chronic illness—including obesity—was in fact a social disease that needed a social cure.

One of the most important elements of this program is tapping into the power of community. I want you to think about weight loss not as a solitary endeavor, but as a team sport.

When we launched the Blood Sugar Solution 10-Day Detox Diet trial, we set up an online community where participants could post their experiences and questions. It was truly amazing to see the participants supporting each other in very personal and profound ways. They shared cooking tips, swapped strategies, lent support when someone was struggling, and cheered each other's successes.

Clearly, social support makes a huge difference. That's why, as part of your Prep Phase, I strongly encourage you to find a buddy, friend, partner, work friend, or faith-based community member to do this program with. Even better, find a group of six to eight people and do this together. You can form a private Facebook group, or meet in person at the beginning, middle, and end, or get together every night for fifteen minutes on Google Hangouts or Skype and check in with each other to share ideas, challenges, and encouragement.

On the 10-Day Detox Diet website (www.10daydetox.com/resources), you can get a full set of instructions and options for how to create and run a group, and community-building tools. You can even join the Blood Sugar Solution 10-Day Detox Diet online course to get daily tools, resources, coaching, and interactive support from me and my nutrition and life coaches.

WHAT YOU CAN EXPECT

During the 10-Day Detox trial program, participants lost an average of 8 pounds (3.5 kg) and 3.4 percent of their body weight (these are the averages; some participants lost as much as 25 pounds or 11 kg!). They lost up to 10 inches around their waist, up to 11 inches around their hips, and their BMI dropped an average of 1.4 points. The average drop in fasting blood sugar was 18 points. The average blood pressure dropped 10 points. But more importantly, people felt better, and many chronic symptoms and conditions resolved.

We had the participants rate and track their overall symptoms, just as you did in the Toxicity Questionnaire on pages 5–7. In ten days, their overall score went down an average of 62 percent. No drug can come close to reducing all those symptoms in that short a time! This is why I say food is medicine and that what you put at the end of your fork is more powerful than anything you will ever find inside a prescription bottle.

TRACKING YOUR RESULTS

The key to believing is measuring your results. The proof is in the numbers! I'm simply going to ask you to track your results at the beginning, through-out, and at the end of the

> I loved tracking my results! It was amazing to see the instant blood sugar corrections and see my waist and hips shrink in only ten days.
>
> — TERRI FRIEDMAN

ten days, and you'll see for yourself the miraculous changes in your own body.

During the Prep Phase, I will give you instructions for exactly what measurements to take. You want to get a baseline of all measurements for comparison.

Then, every morning throughout the program, I'll remind you to take your measurements and stats and record them in your Detox Journal to track your progress. (See page 106 for information about the Detox Journal, or you can go to www.10daydetox.com/resources to use our online tools for tracking all your scores, measurements, vital stats, and daily experiences and feelings through journaling.)

Each evening, you'll record what you ate, how much exercise you did, the number of hours you slept, how many minutes that day you dedicated to the prescribed relaxation techniques. Research shows that people who write down what they do lose twice as much weight as those who don't. Bottom line: Tracking what you're doing creates results. And if you continue to track your results after the 10 Day Detox, you will enhance and extend your results.

TEST YOURSELF

While measuring your blood sugar is optional before, during, and after the 10-Day Detox, I highly recommend it. Many people think you have to be a diabetic to check your blood sugar. Not so. In fact, I think it is a simple, great way for everyone to see how their body responds to what they eat. It will give you immediate and direct feedback about how dramatically and quickly your body responds to the right information in diet and lifestyle.

Some of you may already have a glucose meter and know how to test your blood sugar. Others may want to get a meter at their local drugstore. The newer ones are easy to use, and you can always ask your pharmacist to show you how. I like the ACCU-CHEK Aviva Blood Glucose Meter with Strips, which includes a few test strips (you may need extra).

Here is the protocol I recommend for testing:

- Measure your fasting blood sugar daily, first thing in the morning before breakfast. Ideally, your fasting blood sugar should be between 70 and 80 mg/dl.
- Measure your blood sugar two hours after breakfast and two hours after dinner. Ideally, your two-hour sugars should never go over 120 mg/dl. If they go over 140 mg/dl, you have pre-diabetes. If they go over 200 mg/dl, you have type 2 diabetes. Technically, this is after a 75-gram glucose load, but if they go this high on the plan, you definitely have a problem. Pay attention to how they change depending on what you eat.

GET TESTED BY YOUR DOCTOR

Lastly, I strongly encourage you to consider getting basic lab tests done before and after the program. These would include:

- Insulin response test, which is like a two-hour glucose tolerance test but measures insulin as well. It is done by measuring both insulin and glucose, fasting and one and two hours after a 75-gram glucose drink.
- Hemoglobin A1c, which measures your average blood sugar over the past six weeks. Anything 5.5 percent or above is considered elevated; over 6.0 percent is diabetes.
- NMR lipid (cholesterol) profile, which measures LDL, HDL, and triglycerides, and the particle number and particle size of each type of cholesterol and triglycerides. (This is a newer test, but I would demand it from your doctor, because the typical cholesterol tests done by most labs and doctors are out of date.) This particular test can only be obtained through LabCorp or LipoScience.

Lab tests can be done through your doctor, at most hospitals or laboratories, or ordered by you through personal testing companies such as SaveOnLabs (www.saveonlabs.com). For more information and detailed explanations for each of these tests, go to www.10daydetox .com/resources.

Part of what you're doing over these ten days is becoming an active partner in your health and weight loss plan, and that includes having a full understanding of your numbers and following them over time. I believe everyone should become empowered to learn about their bodies, interpret their test results, and use that information to track their progress.

REMINDER: CHECK IN WITH YOUR DOCTOR

As I mentioned earlier, I have one strong caution to offer before you get started. The program works so well that your blood sugar and blood pressure can drop dramatically in just a day or two. If you are on medication or insulin, you must carefully monitor your blood pressure and blood sugar and reduce your dose of medication in partnership with your doctor to make sure you don't get into trouble. Having your blood sugar or blood pressure run a little high for a week poses almost no danger (if your sugars are under 300 mg/dl and your blood pressure is under 150/100), but rapid drops in blood sugar or blood pressure can be life-threatening. So please be sure to talk with your health care provider before embarking on this journey.

5

The Two Steps to Detox Success

When I train physicians, I explain that learning the science behind functional medicine is very complex, but practicing it is often very easy. All you do is take out the bad stuff and put in the good stuff, and the body does the rest.

Out with the bad, in with the good: These are the two simple but powerful steps behind the success of the Blood Sugar Solution 10-Day Detox Diet.

Here's the breakdown of what you'll be ditching for these ten days and what you'll be adding in.

OUT WITH THE BAD

What exactly do I mean by the "bad stuff"? The bad stuff is all the toxic foods, drinks, and lifestyle habits that are clogging your system. This list also includes foods that are not necessarily "toxic" but are likely to trigger spikes in your blood sugar, as well as other biochemical disruptions:

- All sugar products or anything containing sugar, including honey, molasses, agave, etc., and all liquid sugars, such as sodas, bottled teas, fruit juices, and sports drinks. This includes all artificial sugars and sugar substitutes. No exceptions, so don't ask!

- Gluten, which is a type of protein found in wheat, rye, barley, spelt, Kamut, triticale, and oats.
- All grains (including gluten-free ones).
- Dairy, including milk, yogurt, cheese, ice cream, butter, cream, and casein (often in nondairy products). People often think dairy includes eggs, but I haven't seen a cow lay an egg recently, have you? You can eat eggs on this program.
- Beans, or legumes (this does not include green beans).
- All processed and factory-made foods.
- All refined and processed vegetable oils.
- Alcohol.
- Caffeine.
- Other stimulants or sedatives. If you are on regular medication, don't cease taking it without an okay from your doctor. If you are on "as-needed" medication, see if you can get by without it or gradually taper off your dose. If you are a smoker, of course you should stop, but this may not be the time. One step at a time, one addiction at a time.
- Media overload, the incessant overexposure to phones, texting, the Internet, social media, and television that stresses our nervous system and often shapes our eating behavior and preferences.

I'll explain why eliminating each of these baddies makes such a huge difference.

Sugar

Tonight I lost a battle but won a war. I was at a party and my nemesis, "The Sweet Tea," cast a spell on me. I was weak. I drank it. It was freaking terrible. I won't beat myself up over my relapse because I now understand exactly what I did for myself over these past ten days. I think I needed this little setback in order to really see and believe I was over the junk. Hello, my name is Jenn and I'm no longer a sugar addict!

— JENN WIELGOSZINSKI

If the idea of giving up sugar makes you feel panicky, you're not alone—but don't worry. I'm going to get you through this much more easily than you think. As one 10-Day Detox participant said on the final day of the program (and hundreds more echoed in agreement), "Ten days ago, I couldn't eat enough sugar. Now I don't even want to look at it!" Again and again they were amazed at how quickly and completely their cravings subsided. The 10-Day Detox is specifically designed to curb even the most stubborn sugar addictions and cravings. People often see a change in their cravings in as few as twenty-four hours after beginning the program.

Gluten, Grains, and Dairy

> I am loving this detox! I feel fantastic…thinner and lighter in my body… and I am sleeping through the night for the first time in years. I usually eat pretty well, but I do include lattes and cheese. I am loving having none of those in my body. I think it was the dairy holding me back from weight loss, and I plan to continue this way of eating beyond the ten days. It is great to be held accountable in this first ten days while the cravings subside.
>
> —KIM SCHEEWE-KIRK

The two most common and harmful food sensitivities are gluten and dairy, which is why they are eliminated from your diet during the 10-Day Detox. Many people do not realize that they have hidden food sensitivities. These are not true allergies, like a peanut or shellfish allergy that makes your tongue swell, closes off your throat, creates hives, and can kill you in minutes. These are more subtle reactions to everyday foods. They occur because of small changes in the intestinal tract from multiple insults (such as too many antibiotics, aspirin, acid-blocking drugs, ibuprofen, stress, infections, or even toxins) that allow food particles to enter our bloodstream and get exposed to our immune system. This condition is called a *leaky gut*. We then create low-grade inflammation in reaction to these foreign food particles, which can in turn create many problems—fatigue, brain fog, headaches, depression, allergies, sinus problems, irritable bowel, reflux, joint pain, skin diseases such as acne and eczema, autoimmune diseases, and more. But this inflammation also causes weight gain by triggering insulin resistance.

Gluten is a protein found in wheat, barley, rye, spelt, and oats. It has been around since we began cultivating grains 10,000 years ago (still relatively new in the human diet). But fifty years ago the type of gluten changed as we created new strains of wheat (genetically altered dwarf strains I call Frankenwheat), and this has created a veritable epidemic of problems, including a 400 percent increase in celiac disease and a dramatic rise in gluten sensitivity, affecting about 8 percent of the population.

This new "improved" wheat triggers much higher blood sugar levels because of the amount it contains of the super-starch called amylopectin A. Today, two slices of whole-wheat bread can raise your blood sugar more than two tablespoons of table sugar can. And the increased number and nature of the gluten proteins trigger more inflammation, which increases your risk of obesity and diabetes. We all love bread, but the stuff we are eating today is a far cry from the more wholesome stuff our ancestors ate, and it is making us inflamed, sick, and fat.

All grains (including breads, cereals, and snacks)—even gluten-free ones—can spike blood sugar and insulin. To break the addiction cycle, we need to shut down insulin production as much as possible.

Dairy is also a problem. It not only causes inflammation, allergies, congestion, postnasal drip, sinus problems, eczema, asthma, acne, and irritable bowel for many, it also causes weight gain by spiking insulin levels. It has been linked to type 1 diabetes and is the number one cause of constipation and intestinal blood loss and anemia in kids. It may be "nature's perfect food," but only if you are a calf and want to grow into a cow. For these ten days, you won't be eating any dairy of any kind.

Getting rid of gluten, grains, and dairy for ten days can have profound effects not just on weight but also on many inflammatory, digestive, mood, and other health problems. Think of it as an experiment. You have nothing to lose but your suffering! You can always reintroduce them carefully after the ten days, and in the Transition Phase, I'll walk you through how to do that. But with this short trial, you will have the opportunity to see how they truly affect you— something you probably have never done before.

Don't be surprised if you not only easily drop weight, but also find that many other chronic health problems and symptoms disappear. Pay close attention; this is the most important thing you may do for your health and well-being.

Beans

These are not necessarily "bad," but the carbohydrates in beans can trigger blood sugar spikes in some, and the lectins (small proteins) in these foods can potentially trigger inflammation and weight gain. After the ten days, some of you may choose to reintroduce beans to see how your body responds, but we're going to leave them out of your diet while you detox.

Processed and Factory-Made Foods

As you already know, if you want to turn off the genes that lead to disease and fat and turn on the ones that lead to healthy weight loss, the key is the quality and type of food you eat. So for these ten days, you're going

> "Day 9: Just at the grocery store. My kids beg for Doritos. My mom insists on ice cream. Me? I pick up almonds. I had to do a quick check in the mirror to make sure I was still me."
>
> —JENN WIELGOSZINSKI

to eat a whole-food, plant-rich diet and eliminate foods that are manufactured or produced anyplace other than the earth and your own kitchen.

That means no chemicals, preservatives, additives, artificial sweeteners, high-fructose corn syrup, hydrogenated fats, or monosodium glutamate. (MSG, often called by other names and hidden in almost every processed food, causes spikes in insulin leading to uncontrollable hunger, cravings, and overeating; see the box on the next page to learn how to identify MSG on labels.) You'll eat only the best-quality foods, rich in vitamins and minerals, fiber, phytonutrients, good proteins, good fats, and good, low-glycemic carbs.

Hidden Names for Monosodium Glutamate, and Foods That Contain MSG

- Anything with the word "glutamate" in it
- Gelatin
- Hydrolyzed vegetable protein (HVP)
- Textured protein
- Hydrolyzed plant protein (HPP)
- Yeast extract
- Glutamate
- Autolyzed plant protein
- Yeast food or nutrient
- Glutamic acid
- Autolyzed yeast
- Vegetable protein extract
- Anything "hydrolyzed"
- Protease
- Anything "enzyme modified"
- Anything containing "enzymes"
- Umami
- Carrageenan
- Bouillon and broth
- Stock
- Any "flavors" or "flavoring"
- Maltodextrin
- Barley malt
- Malt extract
- Natural seasonings

Refined and Processed Vegetable Oils

These include corn, soybean, canola, and sunflower oil, and more. All contain inflammatory omega-6 fats and currently make up 10 percent of our calories. During the 10-Day Detox, you'll stick to extra virgin olive oil or extra virgin coconut butter (also known as coconut oil). Extra virgin olive oil contains polyphenols, which are powerful anti-inflammatory and antioxidant compounds. Olive oil has been shown to reduce the risk of heart disease as much as or more than statins. Coconut butter or oil is a powerful cellular fuel and also contains anti-inflammatory fats such as lauric acid, the same fat found in breast milk. For high-heat cooking, grape seed oil is also safe.

Alcohol

Alcohol is just sugar in a different form. Plus, it impairs your impulse control, so you're more likely to eat more—and to do so mindlessly. It also has more calories per gram than sugar (7 calories compared to 4 calories), provokes a leaky gut, and inflames your liver. While it is not all about the calories, if you have one glass of wine a day at 110 calories each, over the course of a year, that can add up to eleven pounds (5 kg) of weight gain. Starting during the Prep Phase, you'll taper off alcohol and cut it out of your diet for the full ten days.

Caffeine

Some say caffeine speeds up metabolism or the rate of calorie burning, called *thermogenesis*. But so do spicy jalapeños or cayenne pepper. Caffeine is hidden in many soft drinks and energy drinks because it is addictive, so you consume more of the sugary drinks. Caffeine also increases hunger.

The research is a bit mixed on coffee because in some population studies, coffee seems to be associated with a decreased risk of diabetes. But in experimental studies, caffeine and coffee have been shown to impair insulin sensitivity in healthy individuals as well as obese individuals and type 2 diabetics.

In one study conducted at the Department of Human Health and Nutritional Sciences, University of Guelph, Canada, ten healthy participants consumed coffee containing 5 milligrams per kilogram body weight of caffeine with a high-sugar meal. They had a 147 percent bigger spike in blood sugar and 29 percent greater insulin surge than those who drank decaffeinated coffee followed by the same meal.

The study showed that coffee consumption followed by a low-sugar, low-glycemic meal was worse. Those people had a 216 percent greater blood sugar spike and 44 percent greater insulin release than those who drank decaffeinated coffee. Researchers concluded that caffeine significantly impairs blood sugar management and insulin resistance.

Getting off caffeine can release you from cravings and normalize your brain chemistry. The problem with caffeine is that you get a surge in dopamine, the reward chemical, but then it wears off. Even if you don't crave more coffee, you will almost certainly crave more sugar. There is a reason there is something called coffee cake. The Blood Sugar Solution 10-Day Detox Diet is designed to completely free your brain from addictive substances. Because decaf still contains some caffeine, it, too, is off-limits for the full ten days.

I want you to have your body back and see what it feels like. From there, you can decide for yourself what you do or don't want to consume. But give yourself a chance to notice what it feels like to detox fully.

In the Prep Phase, I'll take you through the steps to begin weaning yourself off coffee with a minimum of discomfort, so that by the time you begin the program, you're already reaping the benefits of getting this drug out of your system.

Media Overload

Most of us are completely blasted every day with input from all sorts of places that overwhelm our nervous systems: the news, television, radio, the Internet, smartphones, e-mails, text messages, Facebook, Twitter, Tumblr, Pinterest, Instagram…there seems to be more and more input every day.

While these things are often great sources of information, entertainment, and connection, they also have a dark side. They swallow up our attention and our energy and create subtle but constant stress that distracts us from deep healing.

I recently took a ten-day trek in the Himalayas

> One of the wonderful changes I experienced on this detox was learning how to eat without reading or watching TV. It was so relaxing and a joy to concentrate on the taste, texture, and beauty of the food. It really slowed my eating and caused me to be mindful rather than shoveling in the food, which helped me to eat less.
>
> — DIANA STUEF

of Bhutan and was completely removed from all that stimulation. I noticed a calm, deep peace and a dramatic reduction in anxiety, not to mention better sleep and a greater sense of well-being. Of course, being away from work and in the mountains on vacation was helpful, but it was more than that. I often find myself addictively checking my smartphone for e-mails, texts, news, messages, and it takes a toll on me. It's really another form of addiction. In fact, in the new *Diagnostic and Statistical Manual of Mental Disorders* (DSM-V), "Internet Addiction Disorder" is listed as a "condition for further study." Yikes!

I encourage you to take a media fast—a holiday from all nonessential electronic inputs, including television and radio. Think of this program as a detox not just for your body, but for your mind as well—an opportunity to lose all the mental weight and baggage that gets in the way of noticing what is important and true in life.

IN WITH THE GOOD

Now it's time to add in the good stuff!

Each of the elements in the Blood Sugar Solution 10-Day Detox Diet is included because of its powerful ability to help your body heal, detoxify, and shed excess pounds. This special combination of foods and lifestyle practices is scientifically designed to work synergistically to help accelerate and optimize your results. You'll be adding in these potent healing and detoxifying elements:

- Foods that boost detox pathways
- Foods that reduce inflammation
- Foods that improve gut function
- Foods that balance blood sugar
- Exercise
- Supplements
- Hydration
- Journaling
- The UltraDetox Bath
- Relaxation
- Rhythm
- Sleep

Foods That Boost Detox Pathways

The meals and recipes in this program are specifically designed to flood your body with superfoods and phytonutrients to maximize the detoxification process in every cell. In a healthy body, the process of detoxification runs smoothly. When we are toxic, though, the mechanism for detoxification in the liver gets sluggish, and certain toxins can remain active longer than we want or than our systems can handle. This makes us sick and impedes normal metabolism. It also causes fluid retention, bloat, and puffiness.

If you are overweight, you are toxic by definition because most environmental chemicals like pesticides and plastics are stored in your fat tissue. As you lose weight, you need to flush out the toxins that get released from your fat tissue; otherwise, they can poison your metabolism and impair weight loss.

Certain foods speed up the process of detoxification and allow more effective and efficient weight loss. The foods that help boost these detox pathways are those rich in B vitamins, vitamin A, vitamin C, and anti-

oxidants and special detoxifying chemicals called
phytonutrients that are naturally found in bok choy,
broccoli, Brussels sprouts,
cabbage, cauliflower, cayenne pepper, cilantro, col-
lards, garlic, ginger, kale,
lemon, onion, parsley, rose-

> I know about good foods…I still just ate more bad foods, so the foods weren't working in sync. This time I really understand what different foods do to my body, both good and bad, and that's helping me make informed choices.
>
> —JACKIE WOODS

mary, watercress, and sea vegetables like wakame, arame, and kombu.
Eggs are not a plant food but contain detoxifying nutrients and sulfur.

Foods That Reduce Inflammation

Inflammation is your body's normal reaction to fighting off bacteria or
healing an infection or cut. It's something we can see: the red sore
throat, the swollen sprained ankle, the cut that gets infected and turns
red, hot, and tender to the touch. But the inflammation we're concerned with now is hidden inside and doesn't necessarily hurt. It's your
immune system's way of fighting off bad food, stress, toxins, allergens,
the overgrowth of bad bugs in your gut, and even low-grade infections.

Anything that causes inflammation will, in turn, cause insulin resistance. And we already know that insulin resistance causes your body to
generate belly fat and hold on to that spare tire for dear life. So we're
going to focus on cooling the smoldering fire of inflammation that has
been secretly sabotaging your weight loss efforts.

You're already on your way to cooling off the internal inflammation
by eliminating sugar, refined carbohydrates, trans fats, excess omega-6
fats from processed plant oils, artificial sweeteners, MSG, gluten,
grains, and dairy. To maximize the cooling effect, the 10-Day Detox
contains many foods that are rich in omega-3 fats, such as salmon,
omega-3 eggs, grass-fed beef, chia seeds, hemp seeds, flaxseeds, and
walnuts. Herbs and spices such as turmeric and the whole, real, fresh
foods in the menus and recipes are helpful for cooling inflammation,

especially berries, dark-green leafy vegetables, extra virgin olive oil, healthy fats like those in nuts and avocados, and high-quality protein, such as organic poultry, wild seafood, and non-GMO tofu and tempeh.

Foods That Improve Gut Function

Within our digestive system, we each have 500 species of bacterial bugs that control digestion, metabolism, and inflammation. A whole new field of research has emerged on the human "microbiome" (the community of microbes and their genes within the human gut), and it suggests that your weight may be controlled more by what your bacteria eat than by what you eat yourself.

Different bugs thrive in your system, depending on what you feed them. Eating whole, real, fresh foods enables good bugs to grow. Those good bugs can consume as much as 50 percent of your caloric intake, leaving less food for you to absorb. Good bugs boost your metabolism. Eating junk, on the other hand, causes bad bugs to grow and thrive. And bad bugs produce nasty toxins and gas that cause weight gain, inflammation, puffiness, the dreaded belly bloat, and diabesity.

When you eat the wrong stuff, instead of symbiosis—a mutually beneficial relationship between you and your intestinal flora—you create a harmful imbalance that damages your gut lining, creating a leaky gut. Partially digested food particles and microbial toxins then leak across your gut, triggering an inflammatory response (your body's way of protecting you from these "foreign" proteins). The inflammation, in turn, damages your metabolism, affects how your brain controls appetite, and creates insulin resistance and—you guessed it—weight gain.

The whole-food, high-fiber, low-starch, and low-sugar diet that this detox is based on starves the bad bugs and feeds the good bugs. It contains foods rich in the vitamins and minerals that improve gut function, such as pumpkin seeds and bok choy, which are high in zinc, and arugula, kale, tomatoes, and carrots, which are chock-full of vitamin A. It also contains foods such as chicken, turkey, salmon, onions, and parsley, which contain amino acids and antioxidants that promote healing of the gut lining, as well as probiotics to reduce belly bloat, found in kimchi.

Foods That Balance Blood Sugar

Protein is key for balancing your blood sugar. Each lunch and dinner contains some form of lean (and preferably organic) animal protein, complemented by delicious vegetables.

There is much debate about paleo vs. vegan diets that seems worth mentioning here. While a predominantly plant-based diet (meaning that you are eating a lot of actual plants, not a lot of flours and sugars made from plants) is definitely healthful, a purely vegan diet can be a problem for a lot of people with weight issues. It's not always the case, but I've seen a lot of vegetarians and vegans who have serious health and weight problems because their go-to substitutes for meat are starch: rice, pasta, bread, and other carb-heavy, nutrient-poor foods that, once consumed, turn to sugar in their bodies and drive cravings.

Even other grains and beans can be a problem for some vegetarians because they raise blood sugar and insulin more than animal proteins do. It can be unhealthy unless you really know what you're doing nutritionally. Yes, we absolutely should be eating less factory-farmed meat for the sake of our planet, but animal-based proteins are important for many people. And if they come from sustainable wild or pasture-raised sources, I believe they can be very healthy.

What kind of diet is right for you depends partially on the current state of your health and metabolism. The sicker you are, the less wiggle room you have in terms of the amount of sugar you can safely take in. As you lose weight, your resilience increases, and after the 10-Day Detox you can experiment with grains and beans as protein sources. But if you have significant weight or health concerns, for now, I'd counsel you to steer clear of them.

On the 10-Day Detox, you'll notice that two traditional soy proteins are included: tofu and tempeh. While soybeans technically are, obviously, beans, these two foods are notably lower on the glycemic index and don't cause the same blood sugar spikes that other soy products do.

Nuts and seeds are the exception when it comes to plant protein. They don't raise blood sugar and are a fantastic go-to snack for anyone without nut allergies, especially those with diabesity. Nuts have been proven to reduce the risk of diabetes, improve metabolism, and help with weight loss. They are a great source of protein, good fats, fiber, and minerals, including magnesium and zinc, which are key in reversing diabesity.

Exercise

Each of your ten days begins with thirty minutes of moderate exercise. This can have an extraordinary effect on the rest of your day, jump-starting your metabolic engine and balancing your brain chemistry, blood sugar, and hormones so you make better choices. Exercise reduces cravings and regulates appetite, improves insulin sensitivity, boosts the number and function of your mitochondria (improving your overall metabolism), mobilizes detox pathways to help eliminate weight-causing environmental toxins, reduces cortisol (the stress hormone that promotes belly fat), reduces inflammation, and promotes better sleep. It is the best antidepressant and antianxiety treatment and improves energy, well-being, and self-esteem. Bottom line: Exercise enhances everything you're doing on this program!

> My body has been wanting me to give it the right food and exercise for so long. It is thanking me with seven pounds lost, aches and pains nearly gone, and more energy to exercise!
>
> — TINA PETRY

If you already have a fitness routine, you can continue to do whatever form of exercise you enjoy for those thirty minutes. If up until now exercise hasn't been a regular part of your life, start with thirty minutes of brisk walking—or even slow walking, if that's all you can do. If you can only do five minutes, start with that and do it twice a day and then work up slowly over the week. Walking is easy, it's accessible to almost everyone, and it doesn't require any memberships or fancy equipment. As you get stronger, you can increase your exercise intensity and experiment with other kinds of activities.

Supplements

There is much confusion about nutritional supplements and conflicting reports about their benefits, effectiveness, and even safety. This is unfortunate, because I believe that for the vast majority of us, they are fundamental and essential for human survival and optimal health. In fact, the word "vitamin" is derived from "vital amine"—vital components found in our diet without which we can get very sick or die. Yet 90 percent of Americans are deficient in one or more essential nutrients because most of us live on processed, nutrient-depleted food. In fact, 10 percent of us don't get enough vitamin C to prevent scurvy, a profound nutritional deficiency syndrome first described in sailors who ate no fresh fruits and vegetables, and up to 80 percent have inadequate levels of vitamin D.

Let me explain briefly what vitamins and minerals do. They are not drugs, they do not work like drugs, and they cannot be studied like drugs, which is why you hear so much confusing information in the media about nutritional research. Vitamins and minerals are essential components of our biology that make every chemical reaction in our body function, including metabolism and calorie burning. Each chemical reaction requires a catalyst (an enzyme), and each catalyst has a "helper" or cofactor (coenzyme). Vitamins and minerals are those helpers.

Without optimal levels of vitamins and minerals, your biochemistry doesn't run well. In order to burn calories in your cells, you need vitamins and minerals.

Most of our ideas about nutrients revolve around the minimum amount we need to prevent severe deficiency diseases like scurvy or rickets, not the amounts we need for optimal or enhanced biological function and health.

When it comes to weight loss, nutrients play a critical role. When we are low on critical nutrients, our bodies crave more food, seeking to get those nutrients. We eat more and more processed junk foods, searching for nutrients that just aren't there. We are starving in the midst of plenty—overfed, undernourished, and never satisfied.

When we eat real food, which contains many nutrients, we are more satisfied and eat less. But still, we need a foundational amount of high-quality nutrients to help run our engines. Getting adequate vitamins and minerals helps you burn calories more efficiently, helps regulate appetite, lowers inflammation, boosts detoxification, aids digestion, regulates stress hormones, and helps your cells become more insulin sensitive.

The supplement program for the Blood Sugar Solution 10-Day Detox Diet is designed to be simple and easy to follow, and works specifically to address insulin resistance and enhance the detox process. The recommended supplements include a special superfiber called PGX that soaks up sugar and fat and helps curb appetite, lower blood sugar, and promote weight loss. You'll find a complete list of supplements and why each is important for the detox as well as where to find them on pages 101–3 in the Prep Phase.

Hydration

Many of us are chronically dehydrated and consume caffeinated drinks, which makes us even more dehydrated. Simple hydration has been associated with weight loss and helps maximize detoxification by flushing out metabolic and environmental toxins through your kidneys, promotes healthy bowel movements, and increases energy. That is why it's so important to drink at least eight glasses of water each day during the detox and beyond.

Studies show that simply drinking two glasses of water before you eat can lead to significant weight loss. We often mistake thirst for hunger and eat instead of drink, so keep a big bottle of fresh filtered water with you throughout the day and drink. When in doubt, hydrate!

Journaling

The simple act of writing down your experiences and feelings in an unfiltered way has been proven to reduce stress and double the results of any weight loss or behavior-change program. Journaling is one of the most effective ways to break the cycle of mindless eating and process your thoughts and emotions in a proactive, healthy way rather than stuff them down with bad foods and bad habits. As I say often, a diet of words and self-exploration often results in weight loss. Writing helps us metabolize our feelings and calories better. Plus, it keeps us honest and accountable to ourselves, which is crucial for success.

During the Prep Phase, you'll purchase a blank notebook to use as your official Detox Journal, or get the free downloadable Detox Journal at www.10daydetox.com/resources. Each morning of your ten days, I'll remind you to record your progress, and each evening, you'll have specific questions tied to that day's focus to reflect upon. Please don't underestimate or skip this important part of the program.

Relaxation

"You need to relax."

How many of us have heard that piece of advice? And how many of us have nodded, agreed, and then gone about our crazy lives (and crazy diets), swearing we'll get to it when we have the time?

But if you need some real motivation to take that seriously, consider this: Stress increases your levels of insulin, cytokines (messenger molecules of the immune system that trigger inflammation), and cortisol (infamous for promoting the accumulation of belly fat). Stress also increases your appetite and your carb and sugar cravings, triggering the metabolic dysfunction that leads to weight gain. So if you want to lose weight, start by soothing your stressed-out body and mind.

I have built two key relaxation practices into the Blood Sugar Solution 10-Day Detox Diet: the UltraDetox Bath and the Take-Five Breathing Break.

The UltraDetox Bath combines special ingredients to help destress your nervous system, relax your muscles and your mind, alkalinize and pull toxins out of your body, and promote deep, restorative sleep. The Take-Five Breathing Break is a simple yet powerful technique that has a profound effect on your mind and body. You'll learn the specifics of how and when to do these practices in Part IV, but for now, just remember this: Stress makes you fat, and relaxation makes you thin!

Rhythm

Our bodies are biological organisms, and whether we like it or not, or listen to them or not, they are subject to very specific rhythms. Getting our biology back on track depends a lot on getting the timing right. This includes the time you wake and go to sleep, the time you eat, the time you exercise, and the time you relax.

Simple behavior changes to rebalance your daily rhythms can have surprisingly powerful effects: increased energy, better sleep, weight loss, and more. That is why I encourage you to set a schedule of sleeping, eating, exercising, and relaxing every day during your 10-Day Detox and to stick to it.

The science shows that skipping meals, eating very late, and not having breakfast are all guaranteed ways to screw up your metabolism and gain weight. One major cause of diabesity is night-eating syndrome—bingeing at night or getting up in the middle of the night to eat. It is almost always caused by not eating enough during the day and by resultant swings in blood sugar.

Try to establish regular rhythms for eating, moving, relaxing, and sleeping—and watch your body self-regulate into health and natural weight loss. As an added bonus, when you observe set routines and rhythms, you don't have to waste mental energy constantly planning how and when you're going to do your practices and meals each day!

Eating three meals (and a couple of optional snacks if you're hungry) works to keep your sugar and hormones balanced. Eating early in the day kick-starts your metabolism, allowing it to burn hotter all day. And avoiding food two to three hours before bed prevents you from storing it as fat instead of burning it for needed energy. When you sleep, your body is in repair, rebuilding, and growth mode. But the last thing you want to see grow is your belly. That's why observing a sensible daily eating pattern is important.

Sleep

Sleep deprivation has been associated with many diseases, including obesity. I recently read a fantastic book called *Lights Out: Sleep, Sugar and Survival*, by T. S. Wiley and Bent Formby, which chronicles the rise in disease since the invention of the lightbulb. Once we were able to extend our days via artificial light, we fell out of sync with the natural seasonal rhythms and threw off the balance of our body's primitive sleep patterns. In a nutshell, we could stay up later and longer, so we did, essentially tricking our bodies into believing we were in a perpetual state of summer. Our bodies are biologically programmed to store fat and slow our metabolism to sustain us through food-scarce months of winter, which, for most of us modern-day eaters, never actually come.

If you deprive your body of sleep, it increases levels of the appetite-stimulating hormone ghrelin and suppresses the appetite-controlling hormone leptin. Sleep is a natural appetite suppressant, especially when it comes to sugar.

In my thirties, I worked long hours through the night at the ER and was always craving sugar. Cookies, ice cream—you name it, I ate it to keep myself going. If your body can't get enough energy from sleep, you'll look for it from food. Think about it: When you're tired, aren't you more prone to thinking, "I need to eat something"?

These ten days are a chance to see how powerful an effect getting adequate sleep can have on your appetite and fat-storing mechanisms. I recommend getting at least seven hours (but ideally eight hours) per night. In Part IV, you'll find my favorite tips for getting a good night's sleep.

Let's get you prepped for your 10-Day Detox.

PART III

THE PREP PHASE

6

Getting Started

The key to weight loss and health is planning and preparation. The reality is that many people spend more time planning parties and vacations than planning their health. You have to design your life for success and create an environment that directs you toward the right choices automatically. For instance, if you have nuts in your pantry instead of a sheet cake, you are more likely to make a good choice. Setting up your mind, kitchen, and work or school environment right is essential for long-term health and weight loss.

Before you get started on the Blood Sugar Solution 10-Day Detox Diet, set aside two days to do the necessary preparation. To optimize your results and avoid detours and delays, you'll want to have everything you need ready to go.

There are six simple things you'll do during the Prep Phase:

1. Detox your kitchen.
2. Gather your supplies.
3. Taper off caffeine, alcohol, and sugar.
4. Align your mind and intentions.
5. Measure yourself.
6. Join the Blood Sugar Solution 10-Day Detox Diet online community (www.10daydetox.com/resources).

DETOX YOUR KITCHEN

Up until now, your kitchen may have been under the cruel reign of the food industry. Now's your chance to stage a revolution and reclaim it! We're going to start right here, right now, getting the obstacles to weight loss and health out of your way and transforming your kitchen into a place of true nourishment and healing.

Ideally, on the first day of the Prep Phase, set aside a few hours to detox your cupboards, drawers, and fridge. Start by throwing away any item that falls into the following categories. (If you're not sure whether it makes the cut, it doesn't. Get rid of it. Be merciless!)

- Anything that is not real food (i.e., anything made in a factory that comes in a can, box, or package), unless it is a canned whole food, such as sardines or artichokes, with only a few real ingredients, such as water or salt.
- Any food or drink that contains sugar in any form (including honey, molasses, agave, maple syrup, organic cane juice, and artificial sweeteners), especially any sugar-sweetened beverages or fruit juices.
- Anything that contains hydrogenated oils or refined vegetable oils (like corn or soybean oil).
- Any foods with artificial sweeteners, preservatives, additives, coloring, or dyes—basically, anything that has a label or is processed in any way.

The following items also have to go, but if you feel uncomfortable throwing them away, just put them far out of sight during the detox, as long as you feel you can safely avoid them. You may choose to reintroduce some of these in your transition phase, which you'll read about in Part V:

- All gluten products (including bread, pasta, bagels, etc.).
- All grains (even those that are gluten-free).

- All dairy products (including milk, yogurt, and cheese). You may have these in your house for your family, but even your family may not do so well on dairy. If they are big dairy consumers, it would be wise for all to try going dairy-free for ten days. If you don't want to undertake that and can personally avoid eating or drinking these dairy products, then they can stay.
- All beans.

GATHER YOUR SUPPLIES

Here's everything you'll need to have on hand for the upcoming ten days:

Groceries

Now that you've cleared out your fridge and cabinets, restock them with the whole, real, fresh foods that you'll be eating during the ten days. On pages 257–58 you'll find the 10-Day Detox Staples Shopping List, which includes the essentials I encourage you to have in your kitchen. These nonperishable items will enable you to make a variety of healthy meals, both during these ten days and after. I also recommend reading through, in advance, the 10-Day Detox Meal Plan starting on page 261 so you can choose your meals and shop ahead for the specific ingredients you will need for those recipes.

Many people struggle with the expense of buying whole, fresh, good food. However, if you consider the long-term cost of treating diseases that result from eating processed, toxic foods, not to mention the toll that being overweight takes on your happiness and well-being, you may come to view this differently. I encourage you to take an honest look at how much money you spend every week on coffee, sodas, convenience foods, and takeout. What you learn might surprise you. If you give up that daily latte, you could save almost $1,500 a year. You might start to see other hidden funds, too, that would be far better spent on good food and good health.

Having said that, I have a few secrets for shopping smart on the cheap. Seek out local farmers' markets, where you can find fresh produce for less money, or lower-cost stores like Trader Joe's and shopping clubs like Sam's Club or Costco for vegetables, olive oil, fruits, nuts, canned beans, and fish. You can also think about joining a local food co-op, a community-based organization that supports local farmers and businesses and allows you to order food in bulk at just slightly above the wholesale price. Go to www.10daydetox.com/resources to learn how to find one, or check out www.localharvest.org for sources in your area. The Environmental Working Group created a pamphlet on eating well for less called "Good Food on a Tight Budget." You can get it at www.ewg.org/goodfood.

This is a huge opportunity to make a change not just in your shopping and eating habits, but in your family's as well. One detox participant told me her husband gave her grief at first for buying all these "strange" new foods, but by the end, he loved everything she cooked and became her biggest cheerleader.

By doing this detox for yourself, you can stealthily make your family healthier, too. Some members of your tribe may resist, but to the extent that they shift their eating patterns, even a little, they will feel better. I always told my kids that our kitchen was not a restaurant; if they wanted to eat, this was what we were having for dinner. The menu had two choices: take it or leave it. Enlist your family and do the kitchen detox together. Make a game of reading labels and finding the toxic ingredients. Providing your family with real food for ten days will give the important people in your life a chance to see what radiant health can look and feel like—and then they can't help but get on board!

> My children are telling me every day that I look great and I look thinner. They ask what we are eating for the diet tonight and they say I am on with the dishes—meaning they love them!
>
> —HELEN ALLEN

UltraDetox Bath Supplies

Here are the ingredients you'll need for ten days of nightly baths (you'll find the exact instructions for preparing the UltraDetox Bath on page 122 in Part IV):

- Epsom salts (approximately 160 ounces total, enough for 2 cups each night)
- Baking soda (approximately 40 ounces total, enough for ½ cup each night)
- Pure lavender oil (one small bottle should be enough; you can find this at most natural food stores)

Detox Journal

Your Detox Journal will be your constant companion throughout the ten days. Purchase a blank notebook or journal that appeals to you to record your results, thoughts, and experiences. Or you can use the online journal at www.10daydetox.com/resources, which provides all the questions for you to write about.

Supplements

I've made it easy to get the exact supplements I recommend to my patients at www.10daydetox.com/resources. You will need to be on the 10-Day Detox Basic Supplement Pack. (Please note that you will need to order these packs one week before beginning the 10-Day Detox, to allow for shipping time). These will be very helpful during the detox but are also great basic nutritional support for most people and are designed to be taken long-term. Or you may find equivalents at your local health food store. I recommend the following (see the chart on page 103 for a quick summary):

- A high-quality multivitamin and multimineral supplement. This contains all the B vitamins, antioxidants, and minerals you need to help run your metabolism and improve blood sugar and insulin functioning.

- 2 grams of purified fish oil (EPA/DHA), an anti-inflammatory, insulin-sensitizing, blood-sugar-balancing, heart-disease-preventing, brain-boosting supplement.
- 2,000 units of vitamin D3, which helps insulin function. Up to 80 percent of the population is deficient in this important vitamin.
- Additional blood-sugar-balancing and 'insulin-balancing nutrients, including (total daily doses) 500 to 1000 micrograms of chromium, 15 to 30 milligrams of zinc, 300 to 600 milligrams of alpha lipoic acid, 500 to 1000 milligrams of cinnamon, and 100 to 200 milligrams of green tea catechins, which are often found combined in special supplements that optimize insulin levels, blood sugar balance, and metabolism.
- PGX (in powder or capsule form)—a superfiber to slow blood sugar and insulin spikes that can also cut cravings and promote weight loss. Take 2.5 to 5 grams just before every meal with a large glass of water. This can be taken in powder form (½ to 1 scoop) or in three to six capsules; the powder form tends to work better. If you have night cravings or night eating, you can also take a dose after dinner.
- 200 to 300 milligrams of magnesium citrate, once or twice a day, if you are experiencing constipation. This is essential to manage constipation, which can be caused by extra fiber such as PGX if you are not used to it. If you don't have a bowel movement once or twice a day, you may feel ill on this program, so be sure to pay attention to how often you are eliminating and do what's needed to enable you to go every day. Magnesium is also the relaxation mineral and helps reduce anxiety, improve sleep, improve blood sugar control, and even cure muscle cramps.

Supplement	Total Daily Dosage
Multivitamin	Take as directed on the label
Purified fish oil (EPA/DHA)	2 grams
Vitamin D3	2,000 IU
Chromium*	500 to 1000 micrograms
Zinc*	15 to 30 milligrams
Alpha lipoic acid*	300 to 600 milligrams
Cinnamon*	500 to 1000 milligrams
Green tea catechins*	100 to 200 milligrams
PGX (powder or capsules)	2.5 to 5 grams just before each meal; optional additional doses taken throughout the day if needed to control cravings
Magnesium citrate	200 to 300 milligrams (2 to 3 capsules) 1 to 2 times daily

* Chromium, zinc, alpha lipoic acid, cinnamon, and green tea catechins are often found combined in a special supplement; check your local health food store.

PGX: The Wonder Fiber

Most Americans don't eat enough fiber. As a species, we have gone from eating almost 100 grams a day as hunter-gatherers to eating 8 to 15 grams a day or less on a processed-food diet. Fiber helps fertilize the good bacteria in your gut, improve your bowel movements, and prevent cancer and heart disease. But it also helps you lose weight. A special superfiber called PGX (polyglycoplex) has been extensively researched over the past few years. A

(Continued)

unique complex of super polysaccharides from konjac root (glucomannan) and seaweed fibers, it slows the rate at which sugar (and fat) is absorbed into the bloodstream, and it has the overall effect of balancing blood sugar and insulin, reducing appetite, and helping with weight loss.

One of my diabetic patients got off 100 units of insulin just by using this special fiber, and another lost forty pounds (eighteen kilos). That is why I recommend taking PGX before every meal during the 10-Day Detox. If you choose to use only one supplement, PGX is the most important for the detox process.

Please note: To ensure that the fiber moves through your system the way it's meant to, it is essential to drink the recommended eight glasses of water each day. Otherwise, you can get constipated. If you tend toward constipation, please see Day 3 (page 141) to learn how to safely clean out your bowels and stay ahead of this problem. The worst thing you can do during the 10-Day Detox is to be constipated. Taking fiber, magnesium, and vitamin C as explained in Day 3 should resolve the most stubborn cases of constipation.

Optional Testing Tools

If your budget allows, I highly recommend obtaining the following testing tools to really get the most out of your 10-Day Detox transformation (see www.10daydetox.com/resources):

- A glucose monitor
- A FitBit Aria Wi-Fi Smart Scale or Withings scale, which uploads your weight, BMI, and body composition directly into your smartphone
- A blood pressure monitor, which similarly uploads your blood pressure privately into your smartphone for ease of tracking
- A personal movement tracker to track your daily activity and sleep, such as the FitBit, UP by Jawbone, Withings Pulse, or Nike FuelBand

Exercise Apparel

I run nearly every day, or as often as I can. I always keep a pair of running shoes and whatever other weather-appropriate clothing I need together in the same place, so that whenever I'm ready to go, so are my supplies. Think about it the same way you think about cooking: Isn't it much easier to line up all the ingredients and utensils you need than to have to run to the store each and every time you want to whip up something? Remember, our goal here is to set you up for maximum success, and human nature dictates that we are more likely to exercise if we've made it easy for ourselves.

Get your sneakers out of the closet, or go buy a pair. Choose whatever clothing you'll be most comfortable in for walking, and make sure it's clean and accessible. Let's get the obstacle of preparation out of the way so that when Day 1 starts, you're ready to lace up and go.

Water Filter and Bottle

The easiest option to ensure that you are drinking clean, pure water is to filter your own with a simple carbon filter (like Brita) and then carry it with you in a stainless steel or glass bottle. You can find these items at most home goods stores, or even at the supermarket.

TAPER OFF CAFFEINE, ALCOHOL, AND SUGAR

The two-day Prep Phase is the official beginning of what I call your drug holiday—those drugs being caffeine, alcohol, and sugar. These may temporarily make you feel energized and alert, but they wear off fast, leaving you needing more or sparking the vicious cycle of crash-and-crave. A few days off that crazy roller coaster and you'll realize just how much these substances were sabotaging your energy, health, and weight loss efforts.

I would suggest tapering off caffeine in stages. Drink half your normal dose the first prep day, half of that reduced dose on the second day, then quit on the first day of the detox. If you're tired, take a nap. Gentle exercise, lots of water, a hot bath, and extra vitamin C (1,000 milligrams twice a day) can help reduce withdrawal headaches. If it's really bad, try 400 milligrams of ibuprofen. (I know, it is a drug, but I am not a big believer in unnecessary suffering, and one dose is relatively harmless.)

> I did not think I could give up coffee and dairy, but feeling better is a good trade-off. I was extremely tired the first few days, but the fog lifted and I began to experience more energy, a clearer head, better concentration, better mood…and of course the added bonus of weight loss.
> — CORI BLACK

On Day 2 of the 10-Day Detox, our focus will be dealing with detox symptoms. Feel free to jump ahead and read the material on pages 139–40 for a little extra support if you need it during the tapering-off phase.

I would also take this time to go off alcohol cold turkey. And stop drinking any sugar-sweetened or artificially sweetened beverages. Now is the time to stop all processed foods, too. Don't taper, just stop. It's like pulling off a bandage; doing it slowly hurts way more. On Day 1, you will stop all sugar and anything that turns to sugar. But start with the liquid death first!

ALIGN YOUR MIND AND INTENTIONS

A revolution in the body starts in the mind. In the past, your weight loss efforts may have faltered not just because of wrong eating habits, but because of wrong thinking, too. We're going to set that right.

During the Prep Phase, your Detox Journal is your lifeline to rooting out the mental obstacles, beliefs, and attitudes that can sabotage your success. The goal here is to bring awareness to what stands in your way and consciously shift your focus to what you want and know you can accomplish.

Set aside some time during these two prep days when you can fully focus, and write what comes to mind in response to the questions below (the key word here is "write"; just mentally noting the answers doesn't hold you accountable or have the same effect). If other thoughts and feelings emerge, write those, too. The simple act of writing down your unedited inner world is transformative.

- Why am I doing this detox? What is my dream for my body and my life that this detox will make possible?
- What are three specific goals I have for these ten days?
- What are the top three things that hold me back from losing weight? (For example, emotional eating, sugar addiction, choosing poor-quality foods, busy life, food pushers who encourage bad habits, fear of failure, fear of success.)
- What beliefs do I have that might be holding me back? ("I've tried before and failed" or "Losing weight is too hard" or "I don't deserve to give myself this much time and attention.")
- What is my relationship with food, and how would I like to nourish myself?
- How does being overweight or sick diminish or detract from my happiness and from my ability to fulfill my life's purpose?
- How do I see my life changing by my learning to properly nourish and take care of myself?
- What positive experiences have I had in the past that resulted from eating well and practicing self-care and nurturing?

The more you can bring to light the obstacles and opportunities that may be hidden in your subconscious mind, the better chance you have of navigating around them. And perhaps even more important, connecting deeply to your purpose and intention will give you an internal boost of motivation that may surprise you.

Really, why are you doing this program? Who is it for? How might your life be different if you created vibrant health?

I have a type 1 diabetic eight-year-old daughter who is also hypothyroid and gluten-free. So I'm well aware of blood sugar. But I never thought I had an issue with it! It just so happened that I got back blood test results the day I started the program that showed my fasting blood sugar was 91—too high for optimal health. I lost four pounds during the detox and three inches from my waist and hips, my BMI went from overweight to a normal 24.7, and my bloating subsided. But what really surprised me was that my fasting blood sugar went from an average of 90 to 78. I realized I had an issue with all my "healthy" gluten-free snacks!

I am doing the 10-Day Detox Diet to heal for my daughter. I want her to have a great and healthy relationship with food and nourishment. For her, it's life or death—and now I realize it is for me, too. I'm an older mom and if I want to be around for a long time with a quality life, I need to commit to this level of self-care. I'm doing this for longevity, vitality, and my children.

—TERRI FRIEDMAN

MEASURE YOURSELF

Take the following measurements the day before you start the program and record them in your Detox Journal (or go to www.10daydetox.com/resources to find our online health tracking tools):

- **Your weight.** Weigh yourself first thing in the morning without clothes and after going to the bathroom.
- **Your height.** Measure it in feet and inches.
- **Your waist size.** Using a tape measure, find the widest point around your belly button, not where your belt is.
- **Your hip size.** Again using a tape measure, find the widest point around your hips.
- **Your thigh circumference.** Measure the widest point around each of your thighs.

- **Blood pressure.** This can be done by your doctor or at the drugstore, or buy a home blood pressure cuff (go to www.10daydetox
  .com/resources).

Also, be sure to fill out the Toxicity Questionnaire on pages 5–7. And if you are planning to have your cholesterol profile or basic lab testing done (which I strongly encourage you to do!), now is the time. See page 73 for the specific tests you should have done.

JOIN THE BLOOD SUGAR SOLUTION 10-DAY DETOX DIET ONLINE COMMUNITY

The Blood Sugar Solution 10-Day Detox Diet is more than just a program or a book. It's a community. Remember, losing weight and getting healthy is a social activity! You *can* do the program alone, but if you find a buddy, join or

> I think the best part of the program was having a support group I could check in with several times a day. I only commented two or three times, but it was so encouraging to see how well everyone else was doing.
>
> — ANGELA CHRISTIAN

create a group, or join our online community at www.10daydetox .com/resources, you will not only find support for your journey and friends on the path to help if you have questions or get discouraged, you will get twice the results.

You can also join one of our smaller online support groups or even get online or individual nutrition coaching from one of my personally trained nutritionists. I encourage you to join the Blood Sugar Solution 10-Day Detox Diet Online Course to get all the tools you need and connect to a small group or community online to get daily support.

I am also a strong proponent of life coaching to help you get out of your own way. I have used it successfully for many years to help me grow and change behaviors that prevented me from thriving. You can access all these resources at www.10daydetox.com/resources.

A SPECIAL REQUEST FROM ME TO YOU

As you embark on this exciting journey, I encourage you to carve out these ten days as a retreat. How often do you get to do this? Think of it as a gift to yourself—an opportunity to take a health holiday and rest. Un-junk your body, un-junk your mind, un-junk your space, un-junk your life. It's so easy to get sucked up in the chaos of everyday life, so take this time as a personal retreat, knowing that it will radically transform your body.

CHECKLIST FOR THE PREP PHASE

- Do your kitchen detox. Set aside a few hours and go for it!
- Review the 10-Day Detox Staples Shopping List, read through the meal plan to choose your meals, and purchase ingredients for the upcoming days.
- Purchase your supplements if you haven't already.
- Buy the ingredients for the UltraDetox Bath.
- Get a simple carbon water filter and a stainless steel or glass bottle to carry with you.
- Quit alcohol and all liquid sugars (beverages and juices) cold turkey.
- Taper off caffeine, processed foods, and other forms of sugar.
- Get your walking shoes and exercise clothing ready.
- Get a Detox Journal and answer the questions on page 107.
- Take your measurements (weight, height, waist, hips, thighs, blood pressure).
- Fill out the Toxicity Questionnaire on pages 5–7.
- Optional: Get a glucose monitor and learn to use it.
- Optional: Get a FitBit Aria Wi-Fi Smart Scale or Withings scale and blood pressure monitor.

- Optional: Get a personal motion tracker such as the FitBit, UP by Jawbone, Withings Pulse, or Nike FuelBand.
- Optional: Consider basic lab testing.
- Join the online community for support while on the program. See www.10daydetox.com/resources.
- Consider nutrition and/or life coaching to support you on your journey at www.10daydetox.com/resources.

PART IV

THE 10-DAY DETOX

7

Your Daily Practices

Your template for the ten days is simple. While the daily to-dos are the same, the recipes and daily theme are customized so you'll know exactly what to cook, eat, and focus on each day. All you have to do is follow each step carefully and the results happen automatically.

YOUR DAILY SCHEDULE

Here is the plan you're going to follow for each of the ten days. I encourage you to do each of these practices at roughly the same time every day, to balance your biological rhythms and help your body heal:

1. Take your measurements and track your results in your Detox Journal or online tracking tool.
2. Walk (or do another form of moderate exercise) for thirty minutes.
3. Take supplements as directed.
4. Make your Breakfast Detox Shake (take PGX with a glass of water just before eating).
5. Eat a snack (optional).
6. Have lunch (take PGX with a glass of water just before eating).
7. Eat an afternoon snack (optional).
8. Enjoy dinner (take PGX with a glass of water just before eating).

9. Write in your Detox Journal, recording your experience and answering that day's focus questions.
10. Practice the Take-Five Breathing Break for five minutes.
11. Take your UltraDetox Bath.
12. Sleep for seven to eight hours.
13. Throughout the day: Drink eight glasses of clean, filtered water.
14. Throughout the day: Be mindful of the power of a media fast during the program and limit your use of phone, e-mail, and screen time to essential work or personal activities. I promise the world will still be there when you get back.

THE HEALING COMPONENTS OF THE DETOX

The elements included in the 10-Day Detox are designed to work together to create powerful results. You don't have to believe or understand them—just do them anyway. They work automatically. Once you do them, you will discover their hidden synergistic powers of healing. Here's everything you need to know about how to do each of the practices:

Walking (or Other Exercise)

Do your daily exercise first thing in the morning to jump-start your metabolism and set your day on the right course. If you've never exercised before, start with thirty minutes of gentle walking. If exercise is already part of your life or you feel ready for slightly more strenuous movement, go for it! You might be surprised by how motivated and energized you feel.

Tracking Your Results

Each morning, before your walk and before you eat breakfast, record the following stats in your Detox Journal or online tracking tool. Research shows that the simple act of recording these numbers multiplies your success and increases weight loss:

- Weight
- Waist size (measure at the widest part, around your belly button)
- Hips (measure around the widest part)
- Thighs (measure around the widest part)
- Blood pressure
- Blood sugar (optional; this is done ideally before breakfast and repeated two hours after you've eaten; you can also do it two hours after dinner to see how your meal affects your blood sugar)

Each evening, record the following in your Detox Journal or online tracking tool:

- How much sleep you got the night before and how well you slept (deeply or restlessly)
- What you ate that day
- How many minutes of exercise you did
- How many minutes you spent on the relaxation practices
- Any effects you notice related to any or all of the above

> I never stuck to any other program, but my friend encouraged me to try this, saying that she knew I could do it because I like direction and organization. I'm happy to say that I did stick to it, and it was much easier than I thought! Being accountable with the daily stats was a great motivator.
> — FAY SWITSKY

Supplements

Remember, nutrients grease the wheels of your metabolism, help control your appetite, and accelerate weight loss. Each day take the following supplements as directed in the following quick daily reference chart:

- A high-quality multivitamin and multimineral, daily as directed on label
- 1 gram of purified fish oil (EPA/DHA), twice daily
- 2,000 units of vitamin D3, once daily
- 250 to 500 micrograms of chromium, twice daily
- 15 to 30 milligrams of zinc, once daily
- 150 to 300 milligrams of alpha lipoic acid, twice daily
- 250 to 500 milligrams of cinnamon, twice daily
- 50 to 100 milligrams of green tea catechins, twice daily
- 2.5 to 5 grams of PGX in a glass of water (powder or capsules); take just before every meal
- Optional: 100 to 150 milligrams of magnesium citrate, twice a day to prevent or treat constipation

Of all the supplements, PGX is the single most effective supplement for the detox process, as it inhibits insulin spikes and helps clean out your bowels by increasing the fiber load of your diet (for more about PGX, please see page 103). If you tend toward constipation, be sure to add magnesium citrate as noted above.

Supplement	Daily Dosage
Multivitamin	Take daily as directed, with breakfast
Purified fish oil (EPA/DHA)	1 gram, twice daily with breakfast and dinner
Vitamin D3	2,000 IU daily, once daily with breakfast
Chromium*	250 to 500 micrograms, twice daily with breakfast and dinner
Zinc*	15 to 30 milligrams, once daily with breakfast
Alpha lipoic acid*	150 to 300 milligrams, twice daily with breakfast and dinner

Supplement	Daily Dosage
Cinnamon*	250 to 500 milligrams, twice daily with breakfast and dinner
Green tea catechins*	50 to 100 milligrams, twice daily with breakfast and dinner
PGX (powder or capsules)	2.5 to 5 grams just before each meal; optional additional doses taken throughout day if needed to control cravings
Magnesium citrate	100 to 150 milligrams, twice daily, as needed

* These nutrients can be found combined in a special supplement; check your local health food store.

Breakfast Detox Shakes

The morning Breakfast Detox Shakes spark your metabolic fire to burn more calories during the whole day, accelerating weight loss. They are packed with superfoods, proteins, healthy fats, and phytonutrients that will keep your blood sugar balanced and your energy high throughout the day. Plus, they are very filling and satisfying—no worries here about going hungry. As one 10-Day Detoxer said, "I was able to go all day on the breakfast shake. I had to force myself to have lunch!"

I have included several of my favorite shake recipes in the recipe section. I encourage you to try them all to find the one you like the most. The whole-food protein shake (page 267) is my personal favorite—it tastes yummy and keeps your blood sugar balanced all day.

Meals and Snacks

I liked the idea that I knew just what to eat and didn't have to make complicated choices. Having the plan laid out was wonderful! I shopped for what I needed, had it in the house, and was able to pull it all together. Planning meals has always been stressful for me, but once I saw how easy

(Continued)

119

the meals were to make, it took the stress out of it for me. And it got easier and easier on a daily basis. It boosted my confidence to know I could plan and organize healthy meals much more easily than I thought.

— KAREN COLE

Each day has a specific menu plan laid out for you, to take out the guesswork and make sure you get the right balance of filling and detoxifying foods and nutrients. Here's how your meals will go:

Breakfast: Choose your favorite Breakfast Detox Shake.

Lunch: Every day, you have two Core Plan lunch options: You can choose one of the soups in the recipe section, along with protein; or Dr. Hyman's Super Salad Bar, also in the recipe section, along with protein. Alternatively, you can choose the Adventure Plan lunch option listed for that day.

Dinner: Choose either that day's Core Plan dinner recipe (very simple and easy) or the Adventure Plan dinner recipe (for a little extra fun if you have the time and desire to explore).

Snacks: The morning snack each day consists of a small handful of nuts (ten to twelve nuts), such as almonds, walnuts, pecans, or macadamias. This is optional; you may not need it if you still feel full from the breakfast shake. For the afternoon snack, enjoy any one of the dips and spreads in the recipe section, to be eaten with crudités (sliced raw veggies, such as carrots, cucumbers, peppers, or celery). These dips and spreads can be mixed and matched as you like throughout the ten days. Or you can opt for an afternoon nut snack (instead of the spread and veggies) if you prefer.

As I explained earlier, if you are really pressed for time or don't like the Core Plan or Adventure Plan recipes for that day (though I encourage you to have an open mind and try new things!), you always have the option to prepare instead a very basic protein (chicken, fish, tofu, or lean red meat, though limit red meat to once during the ten days) and nonstarchy vegetables (steamed, sautéed, grilled, or roasted). You get unlimited refills on the nonstarchy veggies and can have as many different types as you want at every meal, such as tomatoes, cucumbers, broccoli, greens of any type, asparagus, and green beans. In Chapter 20, you will find a "Cooking the Basics" section that gives you super-simple methods for preparing these easy proteins and vegetables.

Journaling

Every night, set aside some quiet time to write about your day's experience. How are you feeling? What has excited or frustrated you? What changes are you noticing in your body? In your mood? This is your private time to really let your thoughts and feelings fly—write whatever comes to mind without filtering or holding back! Research shows that writing has significant transformational powers to heal and promote weight loss.

During your nightly journaling, you'll also answer the specific questions tailored to that day's focus. These questions were specifically created to guide your interior exploration to deeper levels and clear away any mental or emotional obstacles that might appear along the path.

Take-Five Breathing Breaks

> I had a very stressful day today, and at one point, I thought I'd just go and get an iced tea. I actually parked in front of the place I get my tea and then thought, "Why am I giving up the progress I have made?" So I just sat in the car for a while and did the deep breathing exercises, then calmly started the car and went back to work. I was so proud of myself.
>
> — ANALYN READER

Remember, stress makes you fat and relaxation makes you thin. Relaxation helps you reset your metabolism and lower cortisol. A conscious, deliberate, focused period of deep relaxation and self-awareness every day can profoundly affect your health and your weight.

Each day, I would like you to take five minutes to sit quietly and practice the following deep breathing exercise:

1. Sit on a chair, or propped up on pillows in your bed, or cross-legged on a cushion on the floor.
2. Close your eyes and your mouth.
3. Breath in slowly through your nose to the count of five.
4. Hold to the count of five and then slowly breathe out to the count of five.
5. Do this for five minutes.

If you do this before each meal, you will destress your nervous system, and your digestion and metabolism will work much better. When you do it before you eat, just do five of these breath cycles. And then watch what happens to your appetite and your relationship to food through this simple act of awareness.

Even if you do this cycle of breathing just five times, you will totally transform your brain chemistry and create a deep sense of calm and well-being. It works every time. And it is available to anyone, anywhere, anytime. If you say you don't have five minutes a day for this important ritual, then I say you seriously need to reexamine your life!

The UltraDetox Bath

> I loved the relaxation part of the program. The UltraBath was glorious...I used candles and soft music. I have never experienced such luxury for myself on a daily basis!
>
> — DORA CONRAD

The UltraDetox Bath combines Epsom salts (magnesium sulfate), baking soda (alkalinizing), and lavender oil (cortisol and stress-reducing aromatherapy). When used every night, this ritual creates profound relaxation and detoxification.

Here's the recipe:

- Heat the water as hot as you can stand it.
- Add 2 cups Epsom salts, ½ cup baking soda, and 10 drops of lavender oil. (Optional: light candles and play soothing music to enhance the experience.)
- Add one stressed human.
- Soak for 20 to 30 minutes.

You will love this relaxing ritual so much you will probably want to continue it long after the detox is over. I take an UltraDetox Bath almost every night. It helps me transition to sleep, undo the hurry and worry of the day, and get the triple benefit of mind and muscle relaxation and whole-body detoxification. I use it when I travel, especially when I get back from a long trip; it is my jet lag remedy. Taking an UltraDetox Bath with your partner creates an even more magical healing time to connect and reset your system.

> I have been married twenty-six years and have seen my husband take less than a handful of baths during that time. He took an UltraDetox Bath every night and loved it. It really helped with our stressful lives.
>
> — CHRIS VAUPEL

Get Your Zzzzs

During these ten days, you want to get a mihimum of seven (but ideally eight) hours of sleep each night. Remember, lack of sleep not only damages your cognitive function and your health; it causes cravings for sugar and carbs. Getting enough restful sleep is a powerful tool for stopping cravings in their tracks and promoting weight loss.

Besides the relaxing UltraDetox Bath and Take-Five Breathing Break, here are some of my favorite tips for winding down and getting to sleep easily:

- **Go to bed and wake up at the same time each day,** to instill a regular rhythm of sleep.
- **Use your bed for sleep and romance only.**
- **Create a clutter-free, soothing, restful environment** that encourages sleep. Your bedroom should be a sanctuary that provides peace and calm at the end of your busy days.
- **Create total darkness and quiet** (eyeshades and earplugs are great tools). Remove or cover any lit clocks or electronic digital displays.
- **Get at least twenty minutes of exposure to sunlight a day,** preferably first thing in the morning. The sunlight enters your eyes and triggers your brain to release specific chemicals, such as melatonin, that are vital to healthy sleep cycles and balanced moods, and that help prevent premature aging.
- **Do not eat within three hours of bedtime.** Eating a heavy meal before bed will lead to a bad night's sleep. Energy will be shifted to digesting your meal instead of the repair and healing that is supposed to take place at night. Eating too late is also a guaranteed way to gain weight, because your body will be inclined to store the meal rather than burn it.
- **Avoid bright, stimulating screens before bed.** They alter your brain's natural sleep chemicals. Don't check e-mail, read on your iPad, or check your phone. Watching television right before bed can also significantly interfere with proper sleep.
- **Take an hour (or at least twenty minutes) of complete wind-down time.** The UltraDetox Bath is great for that. Or try reading something soothing in bed.
- **Write down your worries.** You're already making great use of your Detox Journal, so feel free to use it as needed to unload anything and everything that is causing you anxiety and may disrupt your sleep. Making your to-do list for the next day frees up your mind and helps you move into a state of relaxation.
- **Get a massage or stretch before bed** to relax the body. Or learn a few simple restorative yoga poses. One easy pose involves lying on the floor and putting your legs up against the wall. This type of pas-

sive stretching can help calm your body, quiet your mind, and reset your nervous system. At www.10daydetox.com/resources, you can find many DVDs and resources for learning simple yoga routines. Or better yet, find a yoga class nearby and give it a try.

■ **Warm your middle.** This raises your core temperature and helps trigger the proper chemistry for sleep. A hot-water bottle, heating pad, or warm body can do the trick.

■ **Avoid medications that interfere with sleep.** These include sedatives (which ultimately lead to disruption of normal sleep rhythms), antihistamines, stimulants, cold medications, steroids, and headache medications that contain caffeine.

■ **Use herbal therapies.** Try 300 to 600 milligrams of passionflower (*Passiflora*) or 320 to 480 milligrams of valerian root extract (*Valeriana officinalis*) one hour before bed.

■ **Try other sleep-enhancing supplements and herbs.** You might try 1 to 3 milligrams of melatonin, 150 to 300 milligrams of magnesium, 200 to 400 milligrams of theanine, 500 to 1,000 milligrams of GABA (a relaxing amino acid), 50 to 200 milligrams of 5 hydroxytryptophan, and 365 milligrams of magnolia. All of these supplements are best taken just before bedtime. Start with melatonin and then add magnesium. If you are still not sleeping, then you can add the others. See www.10daydetox.com/resources for good sources of gentle, nonaddictive sleep aids.

■ **Get a relaxation, meditation, or guided imagery CD.** At www.10daydetox.com/resources, you'll find my guided relaxation program called *UltraCalm*, which can help you unwind from stress and prepare your body for rest and healing.

I've never been a morning person. Now I get up early, I'm in the office early…I honestly cannot believe that I'm a morning person! I would hit Snooze for an hour if I could. Now my energy has changed so much that I

(Continued)

> get right up and have consistent energy all day long. I'd always thought I
> was a sound sleeper, but now I actually feel rested in the morning.
> — JACKIE WOODS

Hydrate...Times Eight

Be sure to drink at least eight glasses of clean, pure water throughout
the day to help with appetite control and flush out metabolic and environmental toxins through your kidneys. Try drinking two glasses of
water before you eat; that alone has been proven to help you lose
weight. If you like, you can also drink hot water with a squeeze of
lemon or noncaffeinated herbal teas (hot or iced) such as Yogi tea,
Mighty Leaf tea, or Tazo throughout the day.

Note: It is especially important to drink enough water if you are
taking PGX, to avoid constipation. I cannot stress this enough!

Power Down and Do a Media Fast

Turn off the television.
Silence your smartphone.
Log off the Internet. For
the next ten days, with the
exception of all essential

> I found that a quiet house was a welcome
> peace....
> — DONNA STANFIELD

communication, take a brief break from technology and news input.
Spend time with your family, with your friends, or just immersed in
your quiet thoughts; they are all rich sources of nourishment, restora-
tion, and inspiration. Your mind, sense of well-being, health, and
waistline will thank you.

CHECKLIST FOR THE TEN DAYS

- Take your measurements and record the results.
- Do your thirty minutes of exercise.

- Take your supplements (PGX just before every meal with a glass of water and the rest of your morning supplements just before you eat breakfast).
- Make your Breakfast Detox Shake.
- Follow the daily menu plans for snacks, lunch, and dinner.
- Write in your Detox Journal.
- Practice the Take–Five Breathing Break for five minutes.
- Take your UltraDetox Bath.
- Sleep for seven to eight hours.
- Drink at least eight glasses of clean, filtered water throughout the day.
- Enjoy your media fast.

8

Day 1: Satisfy

One of the most amazing things I have found is I have almost NO cravings for sweets or salty foods like I used to. People at work would bring
cookies, candy, and other treats and I would indulge in them big-time.
In fact, I am ashamed to say I would sneak extra portions back to my
office for later...although they never did last until later.

Since embracing this change, I am able to walk right by the treats and
politely decline them when someone specifically brings them to me.
What a great gift that is! I am not bothered watching my friends eat
things I used to eat, and I don't make a big deal about it with "Oh, poor
me, I can't have that." I honestly just don't have a desire for it anymore.

— ANALYN READER

Welcome to Day 1 of your body revolution!

Here's your checklist of today's to-dos, followed by the complete
menu plan:

Morning:

- Take your measurements and record your results in your Detox Journal or online tracking tool. Also record how many hours of sleep you
  got the night before, and the quality of that sleep.
- Begin the day with thirty minutes of brisk walking or other exercise.
- Just before breakfast, take 2.5 to 5 grams of PGX fiber: 3 to 6 capsules or ½ to 1 scoop of the powder in 10 ounces of water.
- Take the rest of your supplements (see page 118) with breakfast.

- Make your Breakfast Detox Shake (see menu plan below).
- Optional: Enjoy a midmorning snack (see menu plan below).

Afternoon:

- Just before lunch, take 2.5 to 5 grams of PGX fiber with a glass of water.
- Eat lunch (see menu plan below).
- Optional: Enjoy a midafternoon snack (see menu plan below).

Evening:

- Just before dinner, take 2.5 to 5 grams of PGX fiber with water.
- Take the rest of your supplements (see page 118) with dinner.
- Eat dinner (see menu plan below).
- Spend fifteen minutes recording your experience and answering the Day 1 Journal Questions listed on page 134. Write down everything you ate and did today, how you feel, any improvements or changes in your energy and focus, and how these changes make you feel physically, mentally, and emotionally.
- Practice the Take-Five Breathing Break (see page 121) for 5 minutes.
- Take your twenty-to-thirty-minute UltraDetox Bath (see page 122).
- Get seven to eight hours of sleep.

Today's Meals:

- Breakfast: Detox Shake of your choice (page 267)
- Midmorning Snack (optional): 10 to 12 nuts (almonds, walnuts, pecans, macadamia nuts)
- Lunch:
  - Core Plan: Choice of soup with protein (page 273) or Dr. Hyman's Super Salad Bar with protein (page 271)
  - Adventure Plan: Kale and Red Cabbage Slaw with Turkey Meatballs (page 288)
- Midafternoon Snack (optional): Dip or spread of your choice (page 317) with fresh vegetables

■ Dinner:
  ● Core Plan: Grilled Salmon with Onion Marmalade over Greens (page 277)
  ● Adventure Plan: Coconut Curry with Fish or Tofu (page 300)

Note: Remember, when you are pressed for time or just want an ultraquick and easy option, you can always prepare a simple protein and vegetable for lunch or dinner from the "Cooking the Basics" section in Chapter 20.

Today's Focus: Satisfy

Most of us have felt the urge—that unstoppable craving—that drives us to seek out something sweet and devour it in a flash. It's that uncontrollable yen for cookies, cake, or ice cream, or that whole basket of bread calling to you to finish it off. Why does that cookie have such power over you, even though you know it will make you fat and sick?

Because most of us don't control food—it controls us. And as you now know, it is not a sign of moral weakness or lack of willpower. Science shows it is a powerfully hardwired brain response that has us reaching for the bread or cookies. Fortunately, it is a response that can be rewired, and today you've taken the first important step to make that happen.

On Day 1, controlling your appetite and cravings is probably front and center in your mind. It may seem inconceivable to you right now that your cravings can ever subside, or that you can navigate between hunger and satisfaction with balance and grace, because you've never experienced that. You've likely been trying to "conquer" your cravings, but cravings can't be wrestled to the ground with willpower. You really can't let go of your cravings. But you can rewire your biological and neural pathways so that your cravings let go of you, and that is exactly what you are doing with this detox.

There is a real science to being satisfied. Swings in insulin drive your cravings. Sugar or anything that turns to sugar is what drives your cravings. Addictive foods that contain heroin-like molecules from sugar and flour and chemicals (like crisps, biscuits, candy, fast food, soda, and even diet soda) drive your cravings. If you can throw a wrench into that biological cycle of addiction, all of a sudden, you're free. You no longer have to fight to control your cravings, because they simply aren't there. Your appetite is controlled by hormones and neurotransmitters, and those in turn are controlled by what you eat. So creating big shifts in your diet can create big shifts in your brain chemistry and, by extension, your appetite. And the good news is that this shift happens very quickly.

For some of you, cravings will go away immediately. Many of the 10-Day Detoxers wrote in to tell me that they were stunned by how quickly that automatic urge for sugar disappeared. For others, it will take a day or two. How fast your cravings vanish depends on how out of balance your biochemistry and metabolism were to begin with. But if you follow the program, the brain chemistry reset will absolutely happen in a matter of days. This program is scientifically and nutritionally engineered to liberate you.

Besides the biochemical component of addiction, there is an emotional component that can run very deep. For some of us, eating is a powerfully charged activity. This shows up in our relationship to food, in our beliefs and attitudes about food, and in how we use it: as comfort, as drugs, as a way to cope, fit in, reward ourselves, or numb our feelings. These deeper explorations are part of the 10-Day Detox that we'll talk about on Day 5, but feel free to read ahead (see page 158) if the emotional aspect is coming up for you right now.

You'll know if you're having an emotional reaction along with the physical one if you feel overly agitated, panicky, or unable to divert your attention from the foods you're not eating. For extra support with this, I recommend two wonderful books by renowned nutritional psychologist Marc David. *Nourishing Wisdom* addresses the emotional underpinnings of some of our difficulties with food, and *The Slow Down Diet* provides a road map out of the maze of emotional eating. You can also get support from his Institute for the Psychology of Eating (www.psychologyofeating.com).

Regardless of your relationship to food, just stick with this "drug holiday," and see what happens. It might be hard to believe, but one day soon you will be able to stand in a donut or pastry shop and look at the treats with no desire to eat them. They simply stop being attractive. That is when you know you own your body again.

I know it's hard to trust that if you make a few simple changes in when, what, and how you eat, your body will respond without struggle. I'm asking you to jump off a cliff without knowing what's at the bottom. But I have seen the proof of these results in thousands of patients and 10-Day Detox Diet participants. It works. So please have faith in your body's capacity to heal. You have nothing to lose but your cravings! The worst place you can end up is right where you started.

If you haven't already, now would be a great time to check in with the 10-Day Detox community. Read what other people are experiencing so you can see for yourself the miraculous and swift changes that can happen. And in "Strategies for Curbing Cravings" below, you'll find some helpful tips to get you through.

Midway through the detox, I bagged up all the grain products in my home and sent them for donation to a local food shelter. You have no idea how huge that was for me. I'd give up all other foods — toxic or not — before carbs. I've let go of all forms of sugar before, but not carbs. At this moment, there are no carbs (except vegetables) in my house and I feel very peaceful about it. Never in a million years would I have seen that coming.

— ANGELA JANNOTTA

Strategies for Curbing Cravings

■ **FOLLOW THE PROGRAM, to the letter.** The combination of carefully selected foods, schedules, protocols, and special lifestyle practices is scientifically designed to eliminate your cravings.

- **Go cold turkey.** Any little bit of a drug will trigger your brain chemistry. That one cigarette...that one drink...What we're dealing with here is an addiction, and even a small amount of what's controlling you will put you right back in its grasp. Sugar, flour, processed food, alcohol, and addictive additives like MSG all stimulate the pleasure center in the brain. They increase dopamine, which makes us feel happy and alert and energetic. We all love that feeling. It's what cocaine does. It's also what sugar does. Those pleasure centers get stimulated, and that makes you want more of that feeling. And more...and more...and more...

- **Avoid your temptation zones.** Be careful to control your environment and where you go during those first critical days. If you were an alcoholic, you wouldn't go into a bar those first few days (or weeks) after quitting. Until you're in the clear from your initial withdrawal period, just steer around your trigger spots: the vending machines, the convenience stores or fast-food places you pass on your way home, the coworker's desk loaded with candy, the cocktail party table loaded with hors d'oeuvres, etc. Even if this means lying low and postponing some social plans for now, that's okay; this is a temporary hiatus you're taking that will soon allow you to embrace life fully and joyfully, liberated from food tyranny.

- **Power up your day with the right combination of foods.** Eat early and eat right. The right breakfast is key. The reason your Breakfast Detox Shake works is that it's nutrient-dense. It's high in protein, fiber, and healthy fat, all of which change your hormones in a way that cuts cravings. The seeds and nuts contain protein, fat, and fiber, and they are also rich in magnesium, zinc, and selenium. Coconut butter provides sustained fuel that makes you feel full. If you want to beef up your shake even more, you can add a scoop of good protein powder made from hemp, chia, rice, pea, or non-GMO whole soy powder. I drink a shake at 7 a.m. and I'm not hungry until noon.

- **PGX before every meal** absorbs water, makes you feel full, reduces your appetite, and reduces the insulin spike. It's a quick way to shut off those appetite-generating hormones. Remember to always drink it with a full glass of water.

- **Keep the daily rhythm of eating** on roughly the same schedule each day. This keeps your blood sugar and insulin levels more even. Blood sugar highs and lows drive primitive food cravings. If you get famished between meals, that's a sign that your blood sugar is crashing. When blood sugar is low, you'll eat anything. Don't wait until you are starved to eat. Incorporate the optional snacks listed in the meal plan to keep your blood sugar even.

- **Prioritize sleep.** When you don't sleep, the appetite-stimulating hormone ghrelin goes up and the appetite-suppressing hormone PYY goes down. Then you start to use food, instead of sleep, to shore up your energy. Think about it: If you're tired, you're instinctively driven to eat to help you stay awake.

Day 1 Journal Questions

- How am I feeling physically today?
- What thoughts and emotions are present for me today?
- What are my beliefs about my relationship to food? Am I in control?
- What false beliefs might I have about my cravings?
- What would my life look like if I were not addicted to sugar, caffeine, flour?
- How does envisioning that make me feel?
- How can I create new habits that will sustain me?

9

Day 2: Detox

I am fifty-seven years old and morbidly obese. I have lost sixteen pounds in ten days. The first day, I had the mother of all headaches. Second day, only a moderate headache. Third day, I woke up with no headache, and the almost-constant pain in my lower legs was gone. Fourth day, I was able to put on running shoes for the first time in four months. By the eighth day, I wore regular shoes to church for the first time in over a year.

— ROBYN JENSEN

Morning:

- Take your measurements and record your results in your Detox Journal or online tracking tool. Also record how many hours of sleep you got the night before and the quality of that sleep.
- Begin the day with thirty minutes of brisk walking or other exercise.
- Just before breakfast, take 2.5 to 5 grams of PGX fiber: 3 to 6 capsules or ½ to 1 scoop of the powder in 10 ounces of water.
- Take the rest of your supplements (see page 118) with breakfast.
- Make your Breakfast Detox Shake (see menu plan below).
- Optional: Enjoy a midmorning snack (see menu plan below).

Afternoon:

- Just before lunch, take 2.5 to 5 grams of PGX fiber with a glass of water.

- Eat lunch (see menu plan below).
- Optional: Enjoy a midafternoon snack.

Evening:

- Just before dinner, take 2.5 to 5 grams of PGX fiber with water.
- Take the rest of your supplements (see page 118) with dinner.
- Eat dinner (see menu plan below).
- Spend fifteen minutes recording your experience and answering the Day 2 Journal Questions listed on page 140. Write down everything you ate and did today, how you feel, any improvements or changes in your energy and focus, and how these changes make you feel physically, mentally, and emotionally.
- Practice the Take-Five Breathing Break (see page 121) for 5 minutes.
- Take your twenty-to-thirty-minute UltraDetox Bath (see page 122).
- Get seven to eight hours of sleep.

Today's Meals:

- Breakfast: Detox Shake (page 267)
- Midmorning Snack (optional): 10 to 12 nuts (almonds, walnuts, pecans, macadamia nuts)
- Lunch:
    - Core Plan: Soup with protein (page 273) or Dr. Hyman's Super Salad Bar with protein (page 271)
    - Adventure Plan: Bok Choy Salad with Tofu or Raw Almonds (page 289)
- Midafternoon Snack (optional): Dip or spread of your choice (page 316) with fresh vegetables
- Dinner:
    - Core Plan: Grilled Snapper with Salad (page 278)
    - Adventure Plan: Chicken Breast with Ratatouille and Steamed Broccoli (page 302)

Today's Focus: Detox

> The process wasn't easy. I had headaches and joint aches. My sleep was off for a while and the cravings were filling my brain with dangerous "feed me!" messages. But I persevered, and you know what? The messages got quieter. My energy levels rose, and my reflux problems literally disappeared. There's no word I can think of to describe it other than "miraculous."
>
> —JENN WIELGOSZINSKI

This book has the word "detox" in it not by accident. You're here to free yourself from food addiction, and just as with detoxing from any drug, that can create a period of discomfort. These are powerful drugs that have taken possession of your brain chemistry and created biological addictions, and it makes sense that your body would have an equally powerful reaction as you come off them. You are rewiring deeply ingrained chemical and neural pathways, and symptoms may arise as your body cleans house and does its job to restore your health.

The following symptoms are common at the beginning of the program:

- Bad breath
- Constipation
- Achy, flulike feeling
- Fatigue
- Headache
- Hunger
- Irritability
- Itchy skin
- Nausea
- Offensive body odor

- Sleep irregularities (sleeping too much or too little, difficulty in falling asleep)
- Brain fog

These detox symptoms are real, and the process of withdrawal can sometimes be difficult and painful. Detox symptoms often get worse before they get better—that's just part of the process as your body cleans out the drugs and toxins. The more toxic and sick you were to begin with, the more intense the symptoms may be. I know this can be discouraging—you're looking to feel better, not worse! But don't worry; feeling good is just a day or two away. While they may feel uncomfortable, symptoms usually pass within forty-eight hours.

I've found that most people are able to deal better with detox symptoms when they understand why they are happening (and when they believe there is light at the end of the tunnel, which, I promise, there is!). This is your biology at its finest, doing its best work to heal you. One of the reasons detox symptoms occur is because your body created antibodies to fight the foods it doesn't like, and when you stop eating the foods, those antibodies are looking for something to do. So they glom on to one another and form giant immune complexes. These big flashing warning signals tell your body that something bad is happening, and they activate your immune system. Your withdrawal symptoms are your body's way of trying to fight off these antibodies. There is actually a name for this phenomenon: It's called serum sickness.

You've probably been in a low-level funk of feeling crappy all along, perhaps without even realizing it. When we eat junk and sugar, our blood is literally inflamed, toxic, or poisoned. We have just gotten used to it slowly, over time. When you stop eating those foods, your immune system is still activated, and you can feel worse for a few days. It takes that long for the body to flush the effects of the inflammatory and toxic foods out of the system.

Another reason for adverse symptoms like irritability, agitation, or anxiety is a true biological withdrawal from an addictive substance. This is exactly the same syndrome that happens in alcohol, nicotine, or cocaine withdrawal. It even happens in rats addicted to sugar.

Fortunately, it usually takes only those few days for this to pass. I recall a detox workshop I held a few years ago during which, in just five short days, the participants saw radical results from following a protocol much like the one you are following now. The first few days, people were tired, lying on the floor, feeling spacey and out of sorts. But by the fifth day, one person was wiggling her fingers, looking at them quizzically. When I asked what she was doing, she said, "This is the first time I haven't had pain in my hands in years." Others found relief from chronic migraines, insomnia, joint pains, irritable bowel, reflux, allergies, and congestion. They lost excess fluid and dropped weight quickly. Many of them left saying they felt like different people.

So I know this from experience: You are only a few days away from feeling well.

And if you follow the strategies and tips I outline below for getting through the initial detox stage, you *will* make it through. Just like your cravings, the detox symptoms will quickly be gone. Hang in there until you get to the other side, because you'll soon feel better than you can imagine.

Strategies for Relieving Detox Symptoms

- **Give yourself some downtime** in the first few days. Rest, take a nap, relax. It's essential for the process. Actively engaging your parasympathetic ("rest-and-relax") nervous system gives your sympathetic ("fight-or-flight") nervous system a break and helps restore your energy, which your body needs to repair itself. Make room for a brief retreat period when you can feel less than great for a couple of days if you need to, and trust that this will pass. Remember, these first forty-eight hours are where a lot of the detox magic happens.

- **Embrace the symptoms as proof that the detox is working.** It may be hard to believe right now, but if you feel lousy, it's a good sign. It means your body is doing what it needs to in order to eliminate the toxins from your body.

- **Flush your system.** Take a sauna, get a massage, do gentle yoga or stretching to flush your circulation and lymphatic system, or take an extra UltraDetox Bath. Any of these increases circulation, reduces inflammation, and thus reduces the achiness and soreness, moves toxins, increases excretion of chemicals, and helps you purify your body.
- **Make sure your bowels are clean and working well.** This will prevent headaches. If you are constipated, please see Day 3 (page 144) for effective strategies to get things moving.
- **Move.** Gentle exercise keeps your circulation going and flushes out all the toxic fluids that build up in your lymphatic system. Even just lying on your back and putting your legs straight up against the wall for twenty minutes can make a huge difference.
- **Take 2,000 milligrams of buffered vitamin C** once or twice a day; this can help relieve symptoms.
- **Drink plenty of fluids.** Be sure to have your minimum of eight glasses of water each day. You can also drink herbal teas if you like (try the Detox Tea from Yogi teas).

Day 2 Journal Questions

- How am I feeling physically?
- What thoughts and emotions are present for me today?
- What detox symptoms (if any) am I experiencing?
- How am I responding mentally and emotionally to these symptoms? (E.g., are they making me feel frustrated, worried, motivated?)
- Can I see that these mental responses are just "the chemicals" talking, and that nothing is actually wrong right now? Or do I still believe that these mental responses are real and justified?
- Can I give myself permission to have a down day—to accept what's happening and allow the process to unfold?
- How can I nurture and support myself through this initial detox process?

10

Day 3: Empty

I thought it was normal to go to the bathroom every two to three days. That's how it's been my whole life. But by changing my diet, adding fiber, and taking extra magnesium, I have gone every single day. For the first time I feel empty and clean and my energy, digestion, and brain fog are so much better. My bloat is gone, I feel lighter and happier. I had no idea that this was what normal felt like.

—SUSAN BERNSTEIN

Morning:

- Take your measurements and record your results in your Detox Journal or online tracking tool. Also record how many hours of sleep you got the night before and the quality of that sleep.
- Begin the day with thirty minutes of brisk walking or other exercise.
- Just before breakfast, take 2.5 to 5 grams of PGX fiber: 3 to 6 capsules or ½ to 1 scoop of the powder in 10 ounces of water.
- Take the rest of your supplements (see page 118) with breakfast.
- Make your Breakfast Detox Shake (see menu plan below).
- Optional: Enjoy a midmorning snack (see menu plan below).

Afternoon:

- Just before lunch, take 2.5 to 5 grams of PGX fiber with a glass of water.

- Eat lunch (see menu plan below).
- Optional: Enjoy a midafternoon snack (see menu plan below).

Evening:

- Just before dinner, take 2.5 to 5 grams of PGX fiber with water.
- Take the rest of your supplements (see page 118) with dinner.
- Eat dinner (see menu plan below).
- Spend fifteen minutes recording your experience and answering the Day 3 Journal Questions listed on page 146. Write down everything you ate and did today, how you feel, any improvements or changes in your energy and focus, and how these changes make you feel physically, mentally, and emotionally.
- Practice the Take-Five Breathing Break (see page 121) for 5 minutes.
- Take your twenty-to-thirty-minute UltraDetox Bath (see page 122).
- Get seven to eight hours of sleep.

Today's Meals:

- Breakfast: Detox Shake (page 267)
- Midmorning Snack (optional): 10 to 12 nuts (almonds, walnuts, pecans, macadamia nuts)
- Lunch:
  - Core Plan: Soup with protein (page 273) or Dr. Hyman's Super Salad Bar with protein (page 271)
  - Adventure Plan: Walnut Pâté with Fresh Tomato Salsa (page 290)
- Midafternoon Snack (optional): Dip or spread of your choice (page 316) with fresh vegetables
- Dinner:
  - Core Plan: Asian-Flavored Chicken Skewers with Wilted Leafy Greens (pages 279–80)
  - Adventure Plan: Grilled Salmon or Tofu Vegetable Kebabs (page 304)

Day 3: Oh happy day! I'm awake and my ankles aren't swollen, nor are my calves. It also appears that my tummy is shrinking. I believe I will become the incredible shrinking woman! I am hopeful my blood sugar will follow suit and drop into normal range soon. This new lifestyle is working. Keep up the race; we are all going to make the finish line!

— WENDY FREEMAN

Today's Focus: Empty

Day 3 brings us to everyone's favorite topic. Yes, that's right: pooping.

It's essential to remove the toxins from your body as you go along. You need to make sure you move your bowels, pee a lot, and sweat. You can detox your diet and your thoughts, but you've also got to clean house, so to speak.

Your body has certain detox systems built in, but if they've grown sluggish, you've got to activate them. This is particularly true of our bowels, which many of us never completely empty. If you are holding on to lots of poop, it can make you toxic, causing everything from gas and puffiness to skin rashes and eruptions.

Even if you are relatively healthy, there may be a surprising (and unhealthy) amount of poop built up in your gut that needs to get flushed out. Here's why: As you detox, your body mobilizes toxins from your cells and tissues and sends them to your liver. Then they get packaged up and excreted through your bile and into your digestive system, and from there, it's your job to make sure they exit your body. Otherwise, they get reabsorbed in a concentrated form, and that can make you feel very sick indeed.

Constipation can make you sluggish, tired, bloated, cranky, and irritable, and can even cause headaches. If you want to feel great, make sure your bowels are moving every day, at least once a day, and preferably more.

Many people have problems with constipation and don't even realize it. I see it routinely: people who go every other day and think that's normal. But it's *not* normal! One woman came to my practice saying that she went regularly…regularly meaning once a week. But if you're moving your bowels any less than once per day, you're constipated. Even if you go every day, and you go incompletely, you are at risk. People who are constipated have higher risks of cancer and even Parkinson's disease. Parkinson's disease is well known to be caused by toxins, be they pesticides or poop!

Constipation is a clue that something's gone wrong in your system. The cause can be diet, especially if you eat a lot of dairy and too little fiber. Dairy can cause lactose intolerance and diarrhea for some, but for others, it causes constipation. In fact, it is the number one cause of constipation in babies. Constipation can happen if you're magnesium deficient, if your gut flora is unbalanced (yeast overgrowth is very common in people with sugar problems), or if you're stressed. Dehydration is a huge cause of constipation, which is why I recommend at least eight glasses of water a day. If you eat fiber like PGX and don't take in enough water, you can get constipated because the fiber turns to a cement-like consistency in your gut. Regardless of the cause, the art and science of moving your bowels is essential for health.

During the detox, you want to be especially vigilant about emptying your bowels at least once a day. These tips and strategies will work for just about anyone. Don't do them all; just start with the first three and then, if you are not going every day and feeling empty afterward, work your way down the list.

Strategies for Easy Elimination

■ **Make sure you drink plenty of water,** to clean out your bowels and flush your kidneys.
■ **Add two tablespoons of ground flaxseeds** per day to your salads, soups, or Breakfast Detox Shakes. Flaxseeds absorb a lot of water and are rich in fiber.

- **Take two 100- to 150-milligram capsules of magnesium citrate** twice a day. You can increase the magnesium dose safely (unless you have kidney disease) to as many as six capsules taken twice per day until you go to the bathroom easily. This is the best way to go regularly. Cut down or stop taking the magnesium if your bowels become too loose.

- **Take 1,000 to 2,000 milligrams of buffered vitamin C** once or twice a day.

- **Take an herbal laxative.** Though this is rarely needed if you follow the strategies above, if you're really clogged up, you can take an herbal laxative such as cascara, senna, or rhubarb (try Senekot or Laxablend by Vitanica, my favorite) before bedtime. Please note: I don't recommend using these regularly, as they create a lazy colon. But it is perfectly fine and safe to use them for these ten days if you need them.

- **If you are really constipated, try liquid magnesium citrate.** Often used to flush out the bowel before a colonoscopy, it's available at your local drugstore, but it's powerful and can really make you go, so be ready and don't leave the house. It usually works in less than four hours.

- **Use a suppository or enema.** If the above methods don't produce results, you can try a Dulcolax or Bisacodyl suppository or a Fleet Enema, available at your drugstore.

- **Get moving to get moving.** Exercise is a powerful bowel stimulant. Daily exercise (see Day 4: Move, page 149) stimulates the colon to do its thing. This is just one of the many benefits of exercise!

- **Sweat profusely at least once a day.** In addition to stimulating the colon, intense exercise allows your body to release toxins through your skin. If your daily exercise routine doesn't cause you to sweat profusely, take a steam or infrared sauna, if possible.

- **If none of the strategies do the trick,** it's time to check in with your doctor to see what else might be going on.

Day 3 Journal Questions

- How am I feeling physically?
- What changes do I notice in my body?
- What thoughts and emotions are present for me today?
- How often do I generally go to the bathroom? (Check in with yourself and take stock of your usual elimination habits.)
- Do I generally drink enough water or get enough fiber in my diet? If not, what changes can I think about making?
- If I am eliminating regularly on this program, how do I feel as a result?

11

Day 4: Move

I started at 209 pounds with high hopes for good health. My initial blood work uncovered that I was anemic, which only gave me more of a reason to eat better. Over the past year, I was constantly out of breath and my heart would pound whenever I tried to do any physical activity. The first two days on the treadmill were tough; it was all I could do to finish a mile in thirty minutes. By Day 10, I was walking at 3 mph and up to 1.5 miles in twenty-five minutes.

I literally watched my health return, and for that I am very grateful. Today I am down nine pounds and four inches off my waist and hips. Simply amazing after only ten days — with no cravings, no lack of food, no deprivation.

— NINA MEFFORD

Morning:

- Take your measurements and record your results in your Detox Journal or online tracking tool. Also record how many hours of sleep you got the night before, and the quality of that sleep.
- Begin the day with thirty minutes of brisk walking or other exercise.
- Just before breakfast, take 2.5 to 5 grams of PGX fiber: 3 to 6 capsules or ½ to 1 scoop of the powder in 10 ounces of water.
- Take the rest of your supplements (see page 118) with breakfast.
- Make your Breakfast Detox Shake (see menu plan below).
- Optional: Enjoy a midmorning snack (see menu plan below).

Afternoon:

- Just before lunch, take 2.5 to 5 grams of PGX fiber with a glass of water.
- Eat lunch (see menu plan below).
- Optional: Enjoy a midafternoon snack.

Evening:

- Just before dinner, take 2.5 to 5 grams of PGX fiber with water.
- Take the rest of your supplements (see page 118) with dinner.
- Eat dinner (see menu plan below).
- Spend fifteen minutes recording your experience and answering the Day 4 Journal Questions listed on page 153. Write down everything you ate and did today, how you feel, any improvements or changes in your energy and focus, and how these changes make you feel physically, mentally, and emotionally.
- Practice the Take-Five Breathing Break (see page 121) for 5 minutes.
- Take your twenty-to-thirty-minute UltraDetox Bath (see page 122).
- Get seven to eight hours of sleep.

Today's Meals:

- Breakfast: Detox Shake (page 267)
- Midmorning Snack (optional): 10 to 12 nuts (almonds, walnuts, pecans, macadamia nuts)
- Lunch:
  - Core Plan: Soup with protein (page 273) or Dr. Hyman's Super Salad Bar with protein (page 271)
  - Adventure Plan: Cod Cakes over Mixed Greens (page 295)
- Midafternoon Snack (optional): Dip or spread of your choice (page 316) with fresh vegetables
- Dinner:
  - Core Plan: Stir-Fry Vegetables with Almonds (page 284)

- Adventure Plan: Bibimbap-Style Vegetables with Egg or
  Tofu in Spicy Chili Sauce (page 310)

Today's Focus: Move

If you've been resisting exercise, you're not alone. Eighty-eight percent of all Americans don't get enough exercise. But your body is growing stronger and healthier with each passing day on the detox, so now is a good time to look inward and explore what might be getting in the way of your getting moving.

So many of us have deeply held beliefs about our ability (or more often, inability) to exercise. Some of these beliefs were hatched early in life, through messages we received. One 10-Day Detoxer named Angela, who had had childhood asthma, had spent her entire young life on the sidelines or relegated to only the most boring of physical activities. While the rest of her class did physical education, Angela was sent alone and humiliated to ride a stationary bike in the athletic training room. She grew up with a belief that "I can't do anything that involves physical activity." Boy, what a bummer of a belief!

By the time she hit her forties, Angela's weight had ballooned to 267 pounds (121 kg). She had lower back pain, knee pain, and swollen ankles, all of which required her to walk up stairs at a creep, pausing with each step instead of taking them one after another. It hurt just to get in and out of a chair. As Angela put it, "I felt physically uncomfortable all the time. Pain and discomfort were my normal—and I was ready to let them go. The exercise part of the 10-Day Detox plan actually concerned me more than the food changes. I knew it all worked together to heal—the food and exercise and other means of self-care. And that's what I wanted, enough so that I was willing to do it."

So Angela shifted her negative belief to "I can find a physical activity that will work for me." She put on a pair of sneakers and for the first time started walking on a regular basis. She stuck to it—no excuses (and this was January in Minnesota!). One step after another, Angela literally walked away from her self-sabotaging beliefs and into a healthier mind-set. Two months later, she wrote to me, "I've still got a long way to go, but for today I feel so much better than I did less than two months ago. My body moves easier and sleeps better. Instead of taking me fifteen minutes to walk from the parking ramp to my office at work, now it only takes ten minutes. I might still be large on the outside, but inside I feel like a supermodel. And with all this energy to burn, I found an exercise I absolutely love—water aerobics. It's so much fun! And it's easy on my joints and has no impact on my asthma. I actually look forward to water aerobics and go three times a week. That is truly miraculous to me."

We are all busy with the demands of work and family, and many of us believe we simply don't have time to exercise. Yet Americans somehow find two spare hours a day to spend browsing the Internet. We spend more time watching cooking on television than we do exercising, and certainly more time watching sports than doing physical activity ourselves.

In my lectures, I often share a funny cartoon. It shows a doctor saying to his patient, "What fits your busy schedule better, exercising one hour a day or being dead twenty-four hours a day?"

When it comes to exercise, little bits do count. Something is always better than nothing! Just the act of taking more steps every day is great. Park farther away from work. Take stairs instead of elevators or escalators. Get a step counter (like a FitBit) and have competitions with friends, family, or coworkers to get to 10,000 steps a day. Or just wear your step counter every day; when you quantify your steps, you're motivated to take more. Find a friend to walk with. Or walk around in circles when you're on the phone!

Strive to fit in exercise wherever and whenever you can. If you look for opportunities, you'll find them. When I'm on the road, I always bring a pair of running shoes so I can go out for a quick thirty-minute run between commitments. I recently found a new seven-minute interval-training workout that I can almost always fit in right when I get out of bed, or before having dinner or going out (see the box on page 154 for more about interval training). It just takes a little planning and intention.

One of the best ways to get yourself moving is to set up the triggers in your life that make it easy to do the right thing. I hate push-ups but realize I need to do them if I want to keep my upper body toned and strong. So I decided to do them right before I get in the shower. Since I shower every day, I am always reminded to do my push-ups, which take less than a minute. Simple, automatic, and easy (well, easy to remember, still hard to do!). It has made a huge difference for me. I started with ten push-ups and can now do forty to fifty at a time.

If Angela can overcome her exercise hurdles, you can overcome yours. All you need are some strategies for releasing your limiting beliefs around exercise as well as real, proven ways to motivate yourself. Read on.

Strategies for Motivation

- **Pair up with a buddy or join a fitness group.** Research has shown that people who are held accountable to others are more likely to stick with an exercise routine. And peer pressure—of the best kind—is a great way to push yourself to do more. I recently went skiing with some friends who took me on a steep double-black-diamond off-trail run—the kind where you needed an avalanche beacon and shovel. Normally I would have said no way, but they assured me I could do it. These are friends I trust, so I took a deep breath and went down…and LOVED it! I was able to do much more than I thought I could with the encouragement and support of friends.

- **Find a reason.** Why are you looking to get in shape? Is it to be able to live pain-free? Is it to be a healthy role model and live a long life for your kids? To feel good about yourself? To fit into your clothes better? Or maybe to look good for someone you love? That's okay! Whatever it takes, connecting to your reasons is one of the greatest motivators for change.

This program is just the kick in the rear I needed to turn my life around. I'm recently divorced, age fifty-two, and would like to meet someone new. However, I know I need to take care of myself and get in shape if I want to attract a man who is fit and active! I'm doing this for myself, first and foremost, but also for my two kids and my future partner. This program made all of this possible…or should I say probable!

—SARAH PETERS

- **Spend some time and effort to find a physical activity that you enjoy.** Personally, I hate going to the gym—I'm much happier playing tennis or basketball, skiing, riding my bike, doing yoga, or doing some other kind of sport. For some people it's dancing; others love power yoga. Find what you love and it'll feel like fun, not torture.
- **Have fun exploring fitness gear.** Take a trip to a sporting goods store and treat yourself to something that feels fun and exciting to you, like new sneakers, a jump rope, an exercise top, or a pair of good swim goggles. Or just pick up a few good fitness magazines to take home and read. You don't have to spend a lot of money to feel inspired.
- **Set up your automatic triggers.** Put your exercise clothes on first thing when you wake up every day, no matter what. Have your workout playlist on your iPod or your DVD ready to go in the DVD player and set a timer to remind you to hit "play." Sign up for an exercise class that you have to show up for at a certain time each day or week. Whatever it takes to make exercise an automatic part of your routine, do it.
- **Set goals.** Sometimes having a goal helps motivate you. Maybe you want to take a special hiking trip with your kids, or do a fifty-mile bike ride, or run a race. Whether it's a 5K walk or an Ironman triath-

lon, having a goal keeps you going. Every summer, I ride around an island off Cape Cod with some friends, and it definitely motivates me to get on my bike and get my butt in shape! Having something to work toward often means the difference between doing something and doing nothing. Plan something, and when that something happens, plan something else. Just keep moving and moving forward. It gets easier and more fun with each accomplishment!

- **Take a little extra time tonight to answer the journal questions** and explore the beliefs and fears about exercise that might be getting in your way. You've come really far these past four days, and now you have a unique opportunity to make some deep and fundamental shifts where it really counts.

Day 4 Journal Questions

- How am I feeling physically?
- What changes do I notice in my body?
- What thoughts and emotions are present for me today?
- What do I believe to be true about myself and exercise?
- What has stopped me in the past from getting in shape?
- What new set of beliefs would serve me better and help me get in shape? (For example, changing your belief that you don't have time into a belief that you can make time for what is important to you.)
- What are the top three reasons I want to get in shape?
- What would my life look like if I were fit and healthy? Is there anything about that image that worries or scares me?
- What kinds of physical activity have I always wanted to try?
- How can I explore these activities? (Hint: Start with baby steps...do some research, get a DVD, try a beginner's class, etc.)
- What practices can I put into place to keep me on track with my exercise routine? (For example, pairing up with a friend for daily walks, committing to a weekly fitness class, or setting small and specific exercise goals to strive toward.)

Ready for More?

At this stage, if you're ready to up the ante on your daily exercise, I recommend incorporating interval training into your routine. Your ability to burn calories is linked to how much oxygen you can consume per minute (referred to as VO2 max). If you have a very high VO2 max, you'll have a very easy time losing weight. How do you get your cells to consume more oxygen? Not by breathing faster, but by making your cells smarter and fitter. You can do this through interval training — exercise in which you're moving alternately fast and slow, or at high intensity followed by low intensity. Interval training can help change your metabolism by making more mitochondria (the little energy-burning factories in your cells).

Interval training also helps you make the best use of your time. High-intensity interval training, or HIIT, involves working at the very top end of your capacity for forty-five to sixty seconds, then recovering for three minutes by walking or a slow jog, then returning to very high intensity for another forty-five or sixty seconds. If you can maintain this cycle for even a few minutes at a stretch, you'll see significant fitness gains very quickly. And you can do it walking, running, biking, jumping rope, dancing, or even swimming. Just focus on getting your intensity up to a 9 on a 1-to-10 scale during the intense intervals, and then allowing your system to recover as much as possible during the rest cycles. And prepare to work up a sweat!

But even if you don't feel up to working out at a high level of intensity, you can still get the benefit of interval training. Generally speaking, any fast/slow/fast/slow routine will help you get far more out of your thirty-minute exercise window than a steady-state workout will. For example, if you're walking thirty minutes, you could do a routine similar to this:

- Two minutes walking at a slow-to-moderate pace to warm up.
- Four minutes walking at a moderate pace.

- Two minutes walking or running at a fast pace (fast enough that you are breathing heavily).
- Continue to alternate four minutes at a moderate pace/two minutes at a fast pace three more times.
- End with three minutes of slow walking to cool down.

I had a patient who was running eight miles a day, and his fitness level wasn't that great. I got him to exercise much less frequently but incorporating fast and slow intervals, and he lost fifty pounds (twenty-three kilos)! That's right: You can exercise less and lose more weight. Studies have shown that people who do interval training can exercise less and yet burn 9 percent more body fat.

If you are in good shape, you might need to work harder to hit the high-intensity level. If you are very out of shape, start slowly. If you have heart disease or diabetes, you should have a stress test or see your doctor before starting a vigorous exercise program. But remember, anybody can start with walking!

There are many different types of interval programs out there that you can explore. A recent study found that you could dramatically improve your fitness and metabolism with a simple seven-minute high-intensity workout. I have been doing it lately; it is hard but worth it. After seven minutes I feel energized and as if I've had a great workout. Go to www.7-min.com for a timer that tells you exactly what to do and when. Many of my readers have had great success with another powerful interval-training program I came across called Pace Express. Go to www.10daydetox.com/resources to learn more about both of these programs.

12

Day 5: Listen

Before the 10-Day Detox program, I had convinced myself that I would never again see the confident, relaxed, positive person who used to live inside my body. Over the last twenty years, food had become my enemy rather than my friend. I didn't even realize the connection between food and my emotions because I believed I was following the principles of a healthy diet...i.e., the food pyramid. In hindsight, I can see that the foods I had been eating left me depressed, irritable, and by midday, lethargic. My attitude went along for the ride, causing me to respond to those around me in a manner of frustration and impatience. After twenty years of trying to "eat right," I had gained sixty pounds and no longer even liked myself. I felt trapped, unlovable, and so very ashamed, stuck somewhere in what I thought was the land of no return.

After the 10-Day Detox, my emotions are miraculously changing. I feel more confident, less anxious, more enthusiastic and energetic. Losing those toxins cleared my thinking. I am now feeling I can find long-term health, recover from those years of being lost in the gloom, and move forward with a positive attitude and resolve. I have lost nine pounds and continue to work toward a healthier lifestyle. I will never go back to my old way of eating. Detoxing my body and mind has recovered the hope that the person I was created to be still resides within my body, and I really like her.

— WENDY FREEMAN

Morning:

- Take your measurements and record your results in your Detox Journal or online tracking tool. Also record how many hours of sleep you got the night before and the quality of that sleep.
- Begin the day with thirty minutes of brisk walking or other exercise.
- Just before breakfast, take 2.5 to 5 grams of PGX fiber: 3 to 6 capsules or ½ to 1 scoop of the powder in 10 ounces of water.
- Take the rest of your supplements (see page 118) with breakfast.
- Make your Breakfast Detox Shake (see menu plan below).
- Optional: Enjoy a midmorning snack (see menu plan below).

Afternoon:

- Just before lunch, take 2.5 to 5 grams of PGX fiber with water.
- Eat lunch (see menu plan below).
- Optional: Enjoy a midafternoon snack (see menu plan below).

Evening:

- Just before dinner, take 2.5 to 5 grams of PGX fiber with a glass of water.
- Take the rest of your supplements (see page 118) with dinner.
- Eat dinner (see menu plan below).
- Spend fifteen minutes recording your experience and answering the Day 5 Journal Questions listed on pages 163–64. Write down everything you ate and did today, how you feel, any improvements or changes in your energy and focus, and how these changes make you feel physically, mentally, and emotionally.
- Practice the Take-Five Breathing Break (see page 121) for 5 minutes.
- Take your twenty-to-thirty-minute UltraDetox Bath (see page 122).
- Get seven to eight hours of sleep.

Today's Meals:

- Breakfast: Detox Shake (page 267)

- Midmorning Snack (optional): 10 to 12 nuts (almonds, walnuts, pecans, macadamia nuts)
- Lunch:
  - Core Plan: Soup with protein (page 273) or Dr. Hyman's Super Salad Bar with protein (page 271)
  - Adventure Plan: Vegetable Rolls with Shredded Chicken and Nut Cream (page 291)
- Midafternoon Snack (optional): Dip or spread of your choice (page 316) with fresh vegetables
- Dinner:
  - Core Plan: Herb-Crusted Chicken Breasts with Roasted Garlic (page 281)
  - Adventure Plan: Roast Fish Casserole with Fennel and Leeks (page 306)

Today's Focus: Listen

Today is a day for tuning in to what's going on in your heart and mind. A few days into a detox, things begin to shift at deeper levels, and it's not uncommon to feel waves of emotions that can catch you off guard. Right around Day 5, we see many 10-Day Detoxers experience profound shifts and gain a greater sense of clarity about their lives, relationships, work, and more.

You might never have done anything like this before—given yourself four days without sugar, processed food, caffeine. As your body heals, certain feelings, sensations, thoughts, and issues that you tended to manage with food may now be exposed. Before this detox, you were pumping up your mood with drugs like alcohol, sugar, and caffeine that kept you artificially stimulated or distracted and didn't allow you to experience what you were really feeling. In fact, you were likely deliberately consuming some of these drugs so that you didn't *have* to feel.

Now, instead of *eating* your feelings, you're *feeling* your feelings. You're no longer under the influence of drugs that make you numb;

you're becoming connected to what's really happening in your life—the good and the bad. And it's important to pay attention. While that can sometimes be painful, it can also be hugely cathartic and life-transforming. It's an opportunity to detox your life and emotions at the very deepest level—to fix the root issues, not just the symptoms. This practice of tuning in to and healing issues in your emotional life has tremendous value for your health. How we feel plays a major role in how we care for ourselves on a physical level, and now is your chance to clean house and set the stage for long-term success.

Maybe you tune in and discover you're sad, or lonely, or afraid. It's useful to pay attention to emotions you may have been stuffing down for years; they can be a wake-up call for changes you need to make in your life. This may seem shocking, but one in four people, for example, have been sexually abused. And many stuff themselves with food so that they don't have to face the feelings associated with that abuse. I have seen this with many of my patients; when we take away the diversion of food, we open up an opportunity for deeper healing by dealing with the root feelings. It is often best to deal with these feelings with the support of a trained therapist or coach who can help sort through this or similar issues.

One patient, Sarah, was in an abusive relationship with her mother and continued to live with her as a fully grown adult. Her mother berated, belittled, and shamed her nearly every day. Sarah had a highly successful career but couldn't get her weight under control. Instead of confronting her mother, she would stuff her feelings down with food and sugar, and she eventually developed type 2 diabetes. The cure for her diabetes, I suggested, might not be diet or exercise, but moving out! Sarah needed to have a real and honest conversation with her mother about the healthier relationship she wanted to build.

When you examine your feelings, you may find that you're feeling guilty for not having taken care of yourself. This is a fairly common emotion that surfaces for people when they wake up to what they have been doing to their bodies. These feelings can be useful because they enable you to see how you may have sabotaged yourself in the past. Even better, they are a sign that you are ready to make better choices. Use these lessons to create a road map of what *not* to do going forward. Just make sure you don't wallow in the feelings of guilt or regret, as they can become just as much of a diversion as the food was. Simply note the feelings and lessons you can learn from them, and move on.

You might also experience positive feelings, and those are equally important to notice. Perhaps you're feeling more awake, alert, and energized. Maybe you're finally free of brain fog, your joints don't hurt as much, or you're just happy that your clothes are fitting better. One 10-Day Detoxer remarked that she spent the day running around after her small child, feeling annoyed that her pants were falling down. Until she realized, "Wait a minute, my pants are falling down...they haven't done that in YEARS!" Acknowledging and celebrating a positive result helps you build motivation and confidence to take on bigger things in your life, so don't pass up the opportunity to acknowledge a job well done.

It's important to stop, pay attention, and tune in to what's happening internally without trying to fix it, control it, or even become attached to it. One of the most powerful skills we can learn is to simply notice and observe our thoughts and feelings without glomming on to them. Feelings change. They shift, often without our having to do anything at all to shift them.

When I was in college, I studied meditation with a Zen master. It was the most basic practice of just sitting, watching my breath, and noticing my thoughts come and go like ripples on the surface of the ocean. It was a powerful experience for me, this simple act of becoming aware that there was something deeper and more essential that made me who I was than my wandering thoughts. By slowing down, breathing, and gently watching the arising and passing of thoughts both pleasant and silly, I began to realize that I wasn't my thoughts or perceptions—there was "me," and then there were "my thoughts," and they were not one and the same. This allowed me to relax more in my life and not hold on to the past or worry so much about the future.

This is an important day to take out your journal and explore your emotions, both good and bad. Write about the challenges, but also celebrate the successes. Take a little extra time today to listen to that inner voice and explore that interior world that has been unconsciously controlling your behavior, and write what you discover. Today is a chance to listen deeply without judgment. This simple practice of awareness writing is something you want to cultivate as you move forward. You have awakened to what's really happening in your body and in your life—you've come too far to bury it all again under food fog.

Today, remember to reach out to others who are following the program; you're not alone in this. This is where your community can really help.

Strategies for Tuning In

■ **Do a basic meditation practice.** This is one of the most powerful things you can do to tap into your deeper spiritual and emotional life (as well as calm your mind, which we'll cover in Day 7). There are many paths of meditation you can try, but here is my favorite basic one, which anyone can do:

1. **Sit quietly in a comfortable place.** Get yourself into a comfortable seated position, perhaps with your legs crossed and your hands resting gently in your lap, or upright in a chair if that's better for you. You want to be able to sit without fidgeting for ten minutes.
2. **Set a timer for ten minutes.** As your practice deepens, try to increase the time by five minutes each day until you reach thirty minutes.
3. **Close your eyes and begin with a few deep, cleansing breaths.**

4. **Turn your attention inward.** Watch your breath as it passes in and out through your nose. Your breath is the steady constant to return to again and again. Don't try to think or not think. If thoughts or feelings surface—which they will—let them. Whatever comes up for you, it's okay. Don't judge or try to shape it. You can live a lifetime in ten minutes, swinging from pleasant, peaceful thoughts and feelings to sad or angry ones. Just let the thoughts and feelings come and go, observing and gently releasing each one as it arises (you can imagine them floating away on a cloud, or vaporizing in the air like a wisp of smoke) and coming back to your breath. You don't need to do anything but listen, notice, breathe, and release.

5. **When the timer goes off, gently and slowly open your eyes.** Spend a few minutes writing in your Detox Journal what arose for you in your meditation practice: what you experienced, how it felt, what insights or shifts you may have had.

Over time you will get calmer and clearer, and this practice will change your brain and how you respond to your own thoughts and feelings. For more information about meditation, go to www .10daydetox.com/resources. My CD *UltraCalm* provides a set of simple guided relaxation, meditation, and imagery experiences that can be very helpful.

■ **Tune in to your body.** Now is a time to pay deep attention to how you feel on a physical level without the sugar and other substances you may have been using to manage your feelings and energy. What is happening to your body? How do you feel from the changes in diet? How are your chronic symptoms? How are you sleeping? How is your energy? Slowing down is key now, so you can really tune in to what your body is telling you. Are the cravings gone or subsiding (by now, they will be for most)? What does that tell you about what you believed to be true for yourself?

▪ **Let yourself be.** Being kind to yourself is key to healing. You don't need to fix anything right now; this is the time to simply notice how you feel. Just listen to what your body and mind are saying and write it all down. The paradox is that the more you accept how things are, the more room there is for them to shift and change. You're opening up to a new awareness of and insight into yourself; trust that you'll continue to make positive changes that will nurture you.

▪ **Extend your journal time tonight as much as possible** and write the answers to the questions below. Recording everything that unfolds for you when it is fresh in your mind is key; while you may think you will remember the powerful epiphanies you have during this awareness meditation, they often fade when we return to the busy-ness of daily life. Write everything down so you capture it fully. Then, in the days and weeks to come, you can go back and reread what you wrote and begin to make whatever changes in your life are appropriate to reflect those inner shifts. The simple act of writing is powerful and healing. Science has shown that twenty minutes of authentic, honest recording of your feelings, thoughts, and emotions can create profound health benefits, including weight loss.

Day 5 Journal Questions

▪ How am I feeling physically?
▪ What changes do I notice in my body?
▪ Have any challenging emotions surfaced for me today? Am I sad, angry, lonely, depressed, frustrated?
▪ Do I have any insight into the source of those challenging emotions?
▪ How have I been using food to avoid dealing with feelings in the past? (To soothe stress, to numb myself, as a reward, etc.)
▪ How can I handle difficult feelings in a more constructive way when they come up in the future? (For example, exercising, journaling, doing a favorite activity, talking to a friend or a professional counselor, checking in with the 10-Day Detox Diet online community,

or just being with people you love can quickly stop a negative emotional spiral in its tracks and elevate your mood. To soothe yourself, reach for what brings you joy rather than for the food.)

- What is one way I could practice that right now?
- Do I need extra help or support to work through these old patterns and beliefs and unconscious behaviors?
- What positive emotions have surfaced for me today? Am I feeling excited, proud, joyful?
- What insight do I have into the source of these emotions? Are they connected to the changes in my body? To my detox experience? How are they affecting my state of mind?
- What strategies do I plan to use to stay connected to the positive emotions I am feeling today? (Hint: Rereading your journal entry to remind yourself of the breakthroughs you had in your awareness meditation today is a powerful tool for grounding yourself in the positive!)

13

Day 6: Think

I finally feel satiated at night, which is unusual for me. There have been evenings in the past where no matter what I put into my stomach, it feels like it's not enough. It is not uncommon for me to have a food hangover in the morning because I have had too much sugar the night before. This program helped affirm that I don't want to treat my body as a garbage disposal. The ideas Dr. Hyman shares about how food speaks to our cells and is used as a drug are powerful. The fact that I can heal myself rather than harm myself with every forkful is something I am more conscious of now.

— HEATHER CUMMINGS

Morning:

- Take your measurements and record your results in your Detox Journal or online tracking tool. Also record how many hours of sleep you got the night before and the quality of that sleep.
- Begin the day with thirty minutes of brisk walking or other exercise.
- Just before breakfast, take 2.5 to 5 grams of PGX fiber: 3 to 6 capsules or ½ to 1 scoop of the powder in 10 ounces of water.
- Take the rest of your supplements (see page 118) with breakfast.
- Make your Breakfast Detox Shake (see menu plan below).
- Optional: Enjoy a midmorning snack (see menu plan below).

Afternoon:

- Just before lunch, take 2.5 to 5 grams of PGX fiber with a glass of water.

■ Eat lunch (see menu plan below).
■ Optional: Enjoy a midafternoon snack (see menu plan below).

Evening:

■ Just before dinner, take 2.5 to 5 grams of PGX fiber with water.
■ Take the rest of your supplements (see page 118) with dinner.
■ Eat dinner (see menu plan below).
■ Spend fifteen minutes recording your experience and answering the Day 6 Journal Questions listed on page 170. Write down everything you ate and did today, how you feel, any improvements or changes in your energy and focus, and how these changes make you feel physically, mentally, and emotionally.
■ Practice the Take-Five Breathing Break (see page 121) for 5 minutes.
■ Take your twenty-to-thirty-minute UltraDetox Bath (see page 122).
■ Get seven to eight hours of sleep.

Today's Meals:

■ Breakfast: Detox Shake (page 267)
■ Midmorning Snack (optional): 10 to 12 nuts (almonds, walnuts, pecans, macadamia nuts)
■ Lunch:
  ● Core Plan: Soup with protein (page 273) or Dr. Hyman's Super Salad Bar with protein (page 271)
  ● Adventure Plan: Chopped Vegetable Salad with Salmon (page 293)
■ Midafternoon Snack (optional): Dip or spread of your choice (page 316) with fresh vegetables
■ Dinner:
  ● Core Plan: Baked Cod with Olive and Caper Pesto (page 282)
  ● Adventure Plan: Almond-Flax Crusted Chicken (page 307)

Today's Focus: Think

Right about now, you're probably starting to feel pretty good (if that hasn't already happened!). The toxins are moving out of your system, so this is a great time to be doing a little of what I call mental flossing. Yesterday you looked at your feelings, and today we're going to look at your thoughts.

You may believe that the results you get in your life come from the actions you take. After all, if you eat cleanly, then you will have a healthy body; if you eat poison, you will have a sick body. But where do these actions originate? What allows one person to succeed at eating well, and another to fail?

Your thoughts are the control center that determines which actions you take. If each time you walk past a bakery, you think, *"Mmm, that smells good. I bet one croissant won't hurt. I've had a rough day, so I deserve a treat,"* then the odds are pretty good that sooner or later you will pop into the bakery and buy that croissant. If, on the other hand, you were to think, *"It just feels so good to be in my healthy body. I have so much energy these days, and am so proud of myself. That vanishes the moment I bite into that croissant . . . not worth it!",* then you are far less likely to eat that croissant. So you can see how important it is that you learn how to design your inner dialogue to work *for* your dreams and not against them.

The first step is to become aware of the thoughts you have on a daily basis that don't work for you. We all have hundreds of thoughts a day, and if we believed every stupid notion we had, we would drive ourselves crazy. Sadly, that is what many of us do, which leads to profound unhappiness and dissatisfaction. But we have a chance today to stop and detox not only from junk food, but also from junk thoughts. We can declutter our bodies *and* our minds.

To do this, take a minute to reflect on one of your dreams for your life. It can be your dream for your body, your career, your relationship with your partner, or any other dream you might have. Think big here.

What is it that you most want for yourself? What will bring you a sense of deep accomplishment and joy?

Next, ask yourself if you believe it is possible to transform that dream into reality. If not, why do you believe it's not possible? What stands in your way? Record exactly what the voice in your head says, down to the exact wording.

For example, when thinking about the obstacles to having a vibrant, healthy body, maybe your inner voice says: "I don't have the right genes to be slim and trim. Everyone in my family is overweight, and there is nothing I can do about it. And besides, even if it were possible to get trim by eating the right foods, I simply don't have time to prepare meals with my crazy work schedule." You've amassed plenty of mental evidence to prove you're right about your genes and your logistical inability to lose weight.

As you read this inner dialogue (otherwise known as the stories we tell ourselves), many of you are likely chuckling. Once we get our inner dialogue out of our heads and onto paper, the thoughts that once seemed so compelling and true often look a little silly. In this purge of our thoughts, we might start to see more clearly our own limiting beliefs about what is and is not possible. The thing about these beliefs is that they are usually not the absolute truth. Most of the time, we've made them up. These stories that we tell ourselves—complete with "evidence" about their accuracy—are what keep us stuck.

There are many ways our thoughts interfere with our staying emotionally and mentally healthy, and these thoughts can take on a life of their own. They loom large in our minds and seem true, even when they aren't, and can have tremendous power over us if we don't examine them.

For example, let's say you believe you can't lose weight because of your genes. Sure, many members of your family may be overweight, but how do you know it's genetic? Have you sequenced your own genome and found the "overweight" gene in there? (Remember, there are only thirty-two obesity genes, and even if you had all of them, that would only account for a twenty-two-pound (10 kg) total weight gain. The habits we inherit from our parents are more important than the genes they bestow on us.) Have you followed the eating plans outlined in this book perfectly and experienced no results (which is nearly impossible!)? Odds are that your belief has very little truth to it. Perhaps you are just holding on to it because it is a convenient excuse not to do the work it would take to get your body healthy. Or your belief may give you a convenient reason not to risk changing your life in a very significant and positive way.

If you have found a belief in your thinking that doesn't work well for you, it's time to gather evidence for a new belief that *does*. In the genetic example, a better belief might be "I can have the body and health I want, no matter what the other members of my family look like." Then you would go out and gather evidence to support that new theory. You would find examples of overweight families that have slim family members. You would think back to a time in the past when you were trimmer. You might even want to prove the new theory correct now by adhering closely to the detox plan outlined in this book, and see what happens.

Where do you self-sabotage? I want to invite you all to take an honest look at where your thoughts and beliefs might have gotten in your way in the past, or even where they might be tripping you up right now. Do you believe it's not possible to be healthy? To be in a happy marriage? To succeed as you want to in life? We're looking to get to the innate beliefs that allow you to be kind to yourself, as opposed to those that fill your mind—and your life—with toxic thoughts, undermining beliefs, and belly-fat-building stress.

Beliefs affect behavior. You think, and you act out of those thoughts. If you have disordered thinking, you have disordered behavior. If you have unhealthy thoughts, they're going to create unhealthy behaviors. We want to flush out the thoughts that are getting in the way of your being fit, happy, and healthy.

Today's strategy is singular: Tune in to your inner dialogue, find those limiting beliefs that hold you back from being the healthiest and most vital version of yourself, and dump them! From there, you can focus on thoughts that work for your dream, not against it. To do this, use the journal questions below—they will walk you through the process of creating a new, empowering inner dialogue.

Consider Life Coaching

In my life, I have struggled with self-limiting beliefs or internal stories about things—rationalizing why I should avoid conflict, or repeating negative thought patterns that keep me stuck and create unhappiness, poor choices, or bad outcomes. That is why I work with coaches in both my personal and my professional life. It's a strategy I often recommend to others who are looking to make significant shifts in their thinking, choices, and behavior.

One of the approaches I've especially liked is the Handel Group coaching model. It has gotten my thinking straight and my actions clear and consistent with my dreams and goals. If you are interested in getting coaching to support you on your journey, give you the kick in the pants you need, and teach you how to get out of your own way, check out http://offerings.handelgroup.com/drhyman.

Day 6 Journal Questions

- How am I feeling physically?
- What changes do I notice in my body since starting the detox?
- What thoughts and emotions are present for me today?
- What is my dream for my health and well-being? (Describe this in as much detail as possible. Articulate your vision of your ideal life, including what you look and feel like, where you will be, what you will be doing, and who you will be doing it with. Dream big!)
- What are my beliefs about my ability to achieve the weight and health goals I've set for myself? Do I think it is possible?

- What do I believe stands in the way of my achieving those goals?
- What mental evidence have I gathered to "prove" that self-defeating story?
- Can I entertain the fact that these beliefs may not be the absolute truth?
- What positive belief would work better for me?
- What examples can I think of that prove the positive belief?
- What new positive, transformative story can I create about where I am headed with my health, weight, and well-being?

14

Day 7: Nurture

Since I can remember, I have found myself eating unconsciously. How did I get to the bottom of that bag of crisps or cookies? Where did that pint of ice cream go? I often eat standing up, or in the car, or while I am doing something else, and then I never really feel satisfied. It's as if I am not really there while the food goes down. The Take-Five Breathing Break ritual of stopping and taking five breaths before every meal changed everything for me. I noticed how I felt and calmed my body down rather than eating in a state of stress (which always makes me eat more). I tasted the food instead of inhaling it and could actually notice when I felt satisfied. Amazing how such a simple exercise could do so much to change my relationship with food. I even noticed throughout the rest of the day how much happier and calmer I felt.

— JENNIFER GENARA

Morning:

- Take your measurements and record your results in your Detox Journal or online tracking tool. Also record how many hours of sleep you got the night before and the quality of that sleep.
- Begin the day with thirty minutes of brisk walking or other exercise.
- Just before breakfast, take 2.5 to 5 grams of PGX fiber: 3 to 6 capsules or ½ to 1 scoop of the powder in 10 ounces of water.
- Take the rest of your supplements (see page 118) with breakfast.
- Make your Breakfast Detox Shake (see menu plan below).
- Optional: Enjoy a midmorning snack (see menu plan below).

Afternoon:

- Just before lunch, take 2.5 to 5 grams of PGX fiber with a glass of water.
- Eat lunch (see menu plan below).
- Optional: Enjoy a midafternoon snack (see menu plan below).

Evening:

- Just before dinner, take 2.5 to 5 grams of PGX fiber with water.
- Take the rest of your supplements (see page 118) with dinner.
- Eat dinner (see menu plan below).
- Spend fifteen minutes recording your experience and answering the Day 7 Journal Questions listed on page 179. Write down everything you ate and did today, how you feel, any improvements or changes in your energy and focus, and how these changes make you feel physically, mentally, and emotionally.
- Practice the Take-Five Breathing Break (see page 121) for 5 minutes.
- Take your twenty-to-thirty-minute UltraDetox Bath (see page 122).
- Get seven to eight hours of sleep.

Today's Meals:

- Breakfast: Detox Shake (page 267)
- Midmorning Snack (optional): 10 to 12 nuts (almonds, walnuts, pecans, macadamia nuts)
- Lunch:
  - Core Plan: Soup with protein (page 273) or Dr. Hyman's Super Salad Bar with protein (page 271)
  - Adventure Plan: Cucumber Salad with Sunflower Mock Tuna (page 294)
- Midafternoon Snack (optional): Dip or spread of your choice (page 316) with fresh vegetables

■ Dinner:
- Core Plan: Roast Chicken Breast with Rosemary (page 283)
- Adventure Plan: Beef with Bok Choy (page 308)

> I could not be more pleased with my progress on the 10-Day Detox. I started out at 202 pounds. I had a lot of edema in my ankles and, quite honestly, was ashamed of my weight and the way it made me feel. I hadn't worn a skirt in years because I didn't want anyone to see my puffy ankles. Even my shoes were tight.
>
> Now, after only six days on this wonderful program, I look and feel great. This morning I weighed 195 pounds. My daughter said I look smaller all over. I have not had one food craving! I don't miss the sugar that I was addicted to or bread or pasta. I feel like I've gotten my life back…I simply feel better.
>
> —DORIS LEE SPRING

Today's Focus: Nurture

When it comes to your health, there is one factor that is more important than perhaps any other. If it is missing from your life, it causes or worsens 95 percent of all illness. It has been associated with dramatic reductions in disease, with longevity, and with weight loss. It doesn't come in a pill, and it can't be found in your doctor's office—because it resides within you.

What is this critical factor that has so much to do with how healthy or sick, fat or slim you are? It is the health of your mind and spirit. In fact, aside from eating breakfast, the biggest predictor of longevity is psychological resilience—being able to roll with the punches that life throws at us. In other words: How we deal with stress dictates the length and, perhaps more important, the quality of our lives.

As I've said before, chronic stress causes your brain to shrink and your belly to grow. That's because the main stress hormone, cortisol, damages the brain, making the memory center (the hippocampus) shrink. Stress shortens our telomeres, the little end caps on our chromosomes. The shorter your telomeres, the shorter your life. And, as you read in Chapter 5, stress also activates a biological response in the body that makes you hungry. It increases your level of insulin and cortisol, sparks an increase in carb and sugar cravings, and at the same time, also increases your body's storage of abdominal fat.

But that's not all. Chronic, unmanaged stress gradually breaks down virtually every system in your body, undermining your immunity and prematurely aging your cells even as it erodes your relationships and your pleasure in living.

The thing about stress is that it just keeps coming around, like the sun. Every day, we are going to be confronted with responsibilities and demands. We have jobs, families, mortgages to deal with. There will be conflicts to face and crises to handle. To some extent, the stuff of modern life makes stress inevitable.

That's why I often tell my patients: "Stress finds you, but you have to go looking for relaxation." Like it or not, it's up to you to find ways to take breaks and manage your stress, for the sake of your health, your sanity—and your waistline!

I noted earlier that there are two parts of the nervous system: the sympathetic and the parasympathetic. The sympathetic nervous system is the part that gets activated in the fight-or-flight response, when your biology charges up to power you through challenges. The parasympathetic nervous system, by contrast, governs the rest-and-relax response—that sense of calm you feel when you can let down your guard, breathe calmly, and just *be*.

The problem is, for many of us, our sympathetic nervous systems are active way too much of the time. It's as if they've gotten stuck in the "on" position. If you want to heal your brain, your metabolism, and your chromosomes, you need to learn how to hit your "pause button" to give your sympathetic nervous system a rest and activate that parasympathetic nervous system instead.

But that doesn't mean sipping a glass of Chardonnay while watching TV or practicing retail therapy. For relaxation to have the restorative effect we're looking for, it has to be active, not passive. Sitting on the couch may be enjoyable, but it's not relaxing. I'm talking about a biological relaxation response in the body that's activated by certain behaviors: breathing exercises, yoga, meditation, massage, even the UltraDetox Bath, all of which encourage deep breathing and profound relaxation of your nervous system.

The trigger for the relaxation response is your breath. When you take a deep breath, you stimulate the vagus nerve—a very special part of your nervous system that helps you calm your mind and turn on a cascade of healing. The vagus nerve runs from your brain through your chest cavity into all your organs, like an octopus stretching out its tentacles to every cell in your body. Your immune cells, your stem cells, and all the other organs and tissues in your body are connected to this nerve.

Stimulating the vagus nerve signals the production of hormones that calm your nervous system, reduce cortisol, help you metabolize your food, boost your brain function, and naturally regulate your appetite. Simply by breathing deeply and activating the vagus nerve, your body starts to boost metabolism and increase fat burning. Pretty amazing.

Science has demonstrated that by stimulating your vagus nerve (which connects directly to your fat cells and the gut), you can trigger all of the following:

- Reduced appetite and food intake.
- Reduced rate at which food is turned to fat.
- Increased metabolism and energy expenditure or calorie burning.
- Increased fat burning in your cells.
- Reduced appetite-stimulating hormones.
- Improved insulin sensitivity.
- Reduced inflammation.
- Increased number of and connections between your brain cells.
- Reduced body weight.

Here's the coolest part: You have the power to stimulate that nerve *anytime you want*. It's low-cost, easy to access, and always available to you. You don't need any special equipment or medication. You can literally change your heart rate, brain cells, brain waves, and weight just by shifting your breath. It's *that* powerful.

Strategies for Self-Nurturing and Stress Release

■ **Remember to do the Take-Five Breathing Breaks.** If you haven't been doing this, it's never too late to start. Begin (or begin again) today.

■ **Find an additional form of active relaxation** that helps you reboot your parasympathetic nervous system. Choose a proven tool that gets you into a profound state of relaxation. Yoga, meditation, tai chi, qigong, biofeedback, playing music—find some activity you can enjoy that also activates the relaxation response. Watching television or reading a book doesn't count. For me, being in nature has a profoundly healing effect. One of my favorite ways to hit the "pause button" is to be outside— by the ocean, in the mountains, by the river, in the forest. Just being outside in the stillness and beauty of nature helps me reset my mind, body, and soul. I'm lucky enough to live in a rural area with mountains, lakes, rivers, and woods, so all I have to do is go outside my front door. But even if you live in a city, go to the roof of your building or into the park and watch the sunrise or the sunset. It has awesome healing powers.

Meditation for Stress Relief

Meditation not only stimulates the vagus nerve and activates the relaxation response—it has also been scientifically shown to make our brains bigger and better. Stress shortens our telomeres (the little caps at the ends of our chromosomes), and this directly impacts our longevity; meditation reverses that. For all these reasons and more, I encourage you to develop even a five-minute daily practice. Also see Chapter 12, "Day 5: Listen." To learn more, go to www.10daydetox.com/resources.

■ **Move your body.** Vigorous exercise is a powerful, well-studied way to burn off stress chemicals and heal the mind. Exercise helps to improve your mood, boost your energy, and reduce overall stress in your body and mind.

■ **Use heat therapy.** Take an UltraDetox Bath or a sauna to turn on the relaxation response. Increasing circulation and increasing body temperature have healing benefits and can reset your autonomic nervous system. Saunas increase heart rate variability, a measure of your stress resilience. The more complex and variable your heart rate, the healthier you are and the greater capacity you have to deal with stresses.

■ **Connect, connect, connect.** Our sense of meaning, purpose, and connection plays a huge role in determining our health and wellbeing. Who do you feel connected to? What gives your life meaning? What were you put on this planet to do? There are so many ways to connect: Spend real and quality time with people you love, join a group of like-minded people, get involved in your community, or volunteer and be of service to others. These are all wonderful ways to nurture yourself and strengthen the bonds of belonging and connection.

■ **Try herbs.** You can use herbs that have been scientifically proven to improve response to stress. Herbs have even been given to astronauts to help them endure the rigors of space travel. I often recommend to my patients the following herbs, most of which can be found in combinations (see www.10daydetox.com/resources):

- 400 to 800 milligrams of ginseng twice a day
- 100 to 200 milligrams of *Rhodiola rosea* twice a day
- 100 to 200 milligrams of Siberian ginseng twice a day
- 800 to 1,600 milligrams of cordyceps twice a day
- 500 milligrams of ashwagandha twice a day

Some of these herbs are available in combination supplements designed to help support your adrenals and create resilience in the face of stress.

■ **Seek out stress-busting tools.** Your smartphone may actually be a biofeedback machine! The iPhone 5 has a heart rate monitor built into the camera. The *Huffington Post* has created an app called *GPS for the Soul*, which has many simple relaxation tools (including one from me) that help you to reset and measure your heart rate variability (the more complex or "variable" your heart rate is, the healthier you are). Meditation, breathing, yoga, and even saunas all increase heart rate variability. This is directly related to your overall health and even to longevity. You can find other stress-busting and biofeedback tools at www.10daydetox.com/resources.

DAY 7 JOURNAL QUESTIONS

■ How do I feel physically?
■ What changes do I notice in my body?
■ What thoughts and emotions are present for me today?
■ What relaxes me most? (Remember, we're talking about active relaxation, not passive.)
■ How can I schedule these activities into my life on a more consistent basis?
■ What events or circumstances in my life usually trigger stress?
■ How do I usually respond to stress?
■ How would I like to respond to stress moving forward?
■ How can I make that happen?
■ How can I remind myself to implement my stress-reducing practice in difficult moments?

15

Day 8: Design

The 10-Day Detox Diet was an eye-opening and life-changing experience for me, to say the least. The plan provided me with just what I needed: a solid blueprint for how to get my health back. There's no word I can think of to describe it other than "miraculous." I lost nine pounds and three inches. My heart isn't pounding out of my chest when I walk up a flight of stairs. My hair doesn't seem to be falling out in big clumps anymore. I have my energy back. I can run and play with my twin toddlers without needing a break. And I can get out of bed in the morning without having to roll out of it!

My husband has been in the army for twenty years and was recently deployed again, and he noticed a change in my voice when he called to check in. He said he's proud of me—that might be the best part of this process. I spend so much time being proud of him for what he does every day, and for him to say the same about me means so much.

How do you thank someone like Dr. Hyman for offering you the opportunity to change your life like this? What can you do to show your appreciation for the new life he's given you? All I can come up with is to continue on this path…to stay healthy and bring your family along on the journey…to continue on with the practices and be a testament to this program. The best thank-you I can think of is to make the most of this gift every day of my life, and that's just what I'm going to do.

—JENN WIELGOSZINSKI

Morning:

- Take your measurements and record your results in your Detox Journal or online tracking tool. Also record how many hours of sleep you got the night before and the quality of that sleep.
- Begin the day with thirty minutes of brisk walking or other exercise.
- Just before breakfast, take 2.5 to 5 grams of PGX fiber: 3 to 6 capsules or ½ to 1 scoop of the powder in 10 ounces of water.
- Take the rest of your supplements (see page 118) with breakfast.
- Make your Breakfast Detox Shake (see menu plan below).
- Optional: Enjoy a midmorning snack (see menu plan below).

Afternoon:

- Just before lunch, take 2.5 to 5 grams of PGX fiber with water.
- Eat lunch (see menu plan below).
- Optional: Enjoy a midafternoon snack (see menu plan below).

Evening:

- Just before dinner, take 2.5 to 5 grams of PGX fiber with a glass of water.
- Take the rest of your supplements (see page 118) with dinner.
- Eat dinner (see menu plan below).
- Spend fifteen minutes recording your experience in your journal. Write down everything you ate and did today, how you feel, any improvements or changes in your energy and focus, and how these changes make you feel physically, mentally, and emotionally.
- Practice the Take-Five Breathing Break (see page 121) for 5 minutes.
- Take your twenty-to-thirty-minute UltraDetox Bath (see page 122).
- Get seven to eight hours of sleep.

Today's Meals:

- Breakfast: Detox Shake (page 267)

- Midmorning Snack (optional): 10 to 12 nuts (almonds, walnuts, pecans, macadamia nuts)
- Lunch:
  - Core Plan: Soup with protein (page 273) or Dr. Hyman's Super Salad Bar with protein (page 271)
  - Adventure Plan: Arugula, Avocado, and Grilled Snapper (page 296)
- Midafternoon Snack (optional): Dip or spread of your choice (page 316) with fresh vegetables
- Dinner:
  - Core Plan: Grilled Pepper Steak and Salad (page 285)
  - Adventure Plan: Chicken Breast Stuffed with Sun-Dried Tomato Pesto, with Sautéed Spinach (page 312)

Today's Focus: Design

Over the past few days, we have examined ways to become healthy from the inside out by addressing your feelings, thoughts, and limiting beliefs. Now it's time to focus on bringing the outside in: on how to design your external environment to support your health so you can continue to make healthy choices easy and automatic beyond these ten days. Changing your behavior is much easier if you set up cues all around you. The less you have to think about it, the easier it is to do. If all you have in the house are raw nuts or crudités for snacks, that's all you will eat. If I was tired or stressed and I had a bag of my favorite chocolate chip cookies in the cupboard, I would eat the whole bag (even though I know better). But if I have to drive ten miles to get it, I won't! It's really as simple as making the defaults in your environment work for you rather than against you. That can be a challenging task when there is a processed-food and junk-food carnival at every corner, but today I'm going to show you how you can set yourself up for success.

In 2009, longevity expert and bestselling author of *Blue Zones* Dan Buettner came to a small town in Minnesota with the purpose of changing the structural design of people's lives to automatically create healthier behaviors. He did this by weaving opportunities to become healthier into the fabric of the community—into schools, workplaces, homes, restaurants, grocery stores, and neighborhoods. He brought together town and community leaders and other experts to rethink the whole problem of health. It was a community-based solution, all about creating simple changes in the environment that led to big changes in health.

Experts on mindless eating (or the study of how unconscious eating habits make us fat and sick) got people to replace their standard-size plates at home with smaller ten-inch ones. Buettner got people to move the junk food up to hard-to-reach shelves in their homes (or to get rid of it entirely) and place fruit and nuts within easy reach. He convinced grocery stores to label and feature foods that helped promote health and longevity. He encouraged businesses to replace donuts, candy, and soda with healthier snacks. Restaurants added healthy options to their menus. Transportation experts designed a sidewalk loop around a lake in the middle of town and encouraged "walking school buses" by getting grandparents to walk their grandchildren to school. Dan and his team of experts encouraged people to form *moai*s, the Japanese word for groups of people who support one another for life (see Day 10: Connect), and walk or exercise together in person instead of "connecting" on social media.

Dan didn't tell people to exercise more, or tell them what to eat. He simply changed their immediate environment. In other words, he restructured the town in such a way as to make it easy for people to do the right thing. As a result, the town saw a 28 percent reduction in health care costs. Kids were no longer allowed to eat in classrooms or in the hallways at school; overall, they saw a 10 percent decrease in body weight. Dramatic changes happened just by altering the infrastructure. It was a groundbreaking experiment that proved the powerful transformational effect of designing your environment for success.

The key to changing habits is to understand how change really occurs. And for the most part, it occurs by design, not by accident or by wishful thinking. It occurs by transforming the unconscious choices we make every day, shifting them so that the automatic, easy, default choices become healthy choices, not deadly ones.

Stanford professor and social scientist BJ Fogg specializes in creating systems to change human behavior. He calls this behavior design. Fogg explains that in order to change behavior, you need three things: the motivation to change, the ability to change, and the trigger to change. If you want to eat a protein-filled breakfast for energy, then you have the motivation. Now you need the ability and a trigger.

For ability, you need to have the ingredients for the breakfast in your cupboard or fridge ready to go and easy to prepare. You might want to measure out the dry ingredients (nuts, seeds, or protein powder) and even put them in the blender the night before. Think low-friction behavior change, so easy you don't even notice it.

Next, you need a trigger. Maybe you put the recipe for a protein shake on your fridge, with a big headline: "EAT THIS FOR BREAKFAST." Maybe you get rid of all the other breakfast options in your house, or put them out of sight so that your hunger becomes the trigger. The point is, you need a catalyst for your new, chosen behavior. You need a built-in nudge that gets you moving in the right direction.

Here's another example: If you are motivated to do chin-ups but never remember and don't have a place to do them, they won't happen. To build in the necessary ability and trigger, you might first purchase a chin-up bar and then install it in your bathroom or bedroom doorway so you see it every time you walk by. With this automatic ability-and-trigger set right in front of you, you will naturally fit in more chin-ups.

Today we're going to focus on redesigning *your* environment to make it easy to do the right thing and create health. Our world is a hostile health environment (we live in a world of Double Gulps and Big Macs at every turn), so we need to create our own "health bubble." I want you to discover how to sync up your motivation, your ability, and the environmental triggers to make doing the right thing automatic.

We're going to design your world to sustain your weight loss long after these ten days are up.

Where is your environment set up to help you stay on track and where does it trip you up? What can you do to make your actions automatic around food, exercise, and stress reduction? Let's take the obstacles out of being healthy and fit!

Below, I've combined the Strategies and Journal Questions sections to help you uncover the obstacles and design your life for optimal health and weight loss. I encourage you to write the answers and plans down in your Detox Journal to cement your intention into commitment. Don't skip this important step—it's the key to your continued success.

Strategies for Healthy Life Design

■ **Organize your kitchen for healthy meal preparation.** You've already done a cupboard and fridge makeover for your 10-Day Detox, and that's a great start. Now take a look around the rest of your kitchen—what would make it easy for you to continue to prepare and eat healthy meals forever? Perhaps you could:

- Clean out your drawers and cabinets so they are free of clutter.
- Make sure you have or buy all the cooking utensils you need to succeed.
- Arrange your pots and pans for easier access.
- Get smaller plates.
- Refresh your supply of spices, condiments, oils, vinegars, and sauces so you can cook anything, at any time, without having to run out to the supermarket.
- Find new recipes online or in cookbooks (such as *The Blood Sugar Solution Cookbook*) and put them in an easy-to-access place so they are ready when you need them.

Identify three things today that would help make your kitchen a source of healthy, nourishing meals. Write your plan for organizing your kitchen, including how and when you will do so, in your Detox Journal as a commitment to yourself. Be as specific as you can—the clearer your plan is and the more accountable you are to a timeline, the more likely you are to make it happen. Your written plan might look something like this:

My Healthy Kitchen Fixes	My Strategy	How/When I Will Make It Happen
Make it easier to find and use my cooking utensils	Organize my pots and pans	This Saturday afternoon
Use smaller plates	Buy an inexpensive set of 8- or 10-inch dishes	Order these online tonight
Find some new recipes that my family likes	Read *The Blood Sugar Solution Cookbook*	Make one new recipe for family dinner on Friday night

■ **Stock your kitchen with the right stuff.** After the detox, continue to fill your cabinets and fridge with all the ingredients and foods that promote health and well-being. You will inevitably open the fridge looking for something when you are hungry, tired, or stressed. So make sure the choices there are going to help you, not hurt you. Arrange the foods so that the healthiest ones are the most accessible and appealing. Cut up veggies and fruit and have them in little glass containers stacked for easy access. Stock healthy snacks (such as nuts, seeds, or grass-fed or organic turkey, beef, or buffalo jerky) so that they are easy to grab on the go when you're in a hurry. Write a list of your favorite healthy go-to foods and snacks in your Detox Journal and commit to keeping them on hand from Day 11 onward.

■ **Make your bedroom a sanctuary.** Compared to your kitchen, your bedroom might not strike you as an influential area for your health and weight loss efforts, but it is. Is your bedroom designed to be a peaceful, stress-free environment that promotes rest? What prevents you from getting a good night's sleep? Look around your bedroom and identify three things you can do to make it a place of rejuvenation. Options might include clearing away clutter, getting blackout shades, getting earplugs or an eye mask, or committing to reading instead of watching television before bedtime (see pages 123–25 for more of my favorite tips for winding down and getting to sleep easily). Record in your Detox Journal these three ideas for designing your restful bedroom and write a detailed plan for how and when you will implement them. Remember, be as specific as you can. Your written plan might look something like this:

My Bedroom Adjustments	My Strategy	How/When I Will Make It Happen
Remove clutter	Clean off my nightstand	Saturday afternoon
Make it quieter	Get noise-reducing curtains	Measure my windows and go to the store next Sunday
Not falling asleep with the television on	Watch the evening news in the living room only	Every night this week

■ **Plan your food in advance.** Think ahead! The goal is to prevent yourself from ending up in a food emergency in which the only thing open is a fast-food restaurant or convenience store. When do you typically get into that type of situation? Is it at 5 p.m. when you're too tired to make dinner? When you're pressed for time between daily commitments and on the run? Identify your top three "trouble time zones" and record in your Detox Journal a corresponding strategy to have food on hand to head off each. Be specific: What foods can you buy or make ahead of time to avert your common food emergencies?

How, when, and where will you purchase or prepare these foods? You can also assemble what I call an Emergency Life Pack (see page 193) to carry with you to ensure you're never stuck without healthy options. Your Detox Journal plan might look something like this:

My Trouble Time Zones	My Strategy	How/When I Will Make It Happen
Mornings when I am rushing to get to work	Make breakfast in advance	Assemble the ingredients for my Breakfast Detox Shake tonight to have ready for tomorrow morning
Sunday late afternoon when I am too tired from weekend activities to make dinner	Prepare a bigger dinner Friday and Saturday nights so I have leftovers on Sunday	This Friday, I will cook _____, Saturday I will make _____, and Sunday we will enjoy the leftovers

■ **Make grocery shopping a weekly ritual.** This goes hand in hand with planning your meals ahead of time. Keep a shopping list at the ready so you can add to it as the week goes along. Choose a specific day and time when you'll shop each week so it becomes an ingrained ritual. Write your plan for weekly grocery shopping in your Detox Journal.

■ **Plant healthy snacks in your environment.** Put raw nuts or other healthy snacks in your glove compartment, desk drawer, purse, or backpack so they are within easy reach and allow you to safely bypass the vending machine or drive-through when you're hungry. Write your specific plan in your Detox Journal for where, when, and what healthy foods you will plant in your environment. Your plan might look something like this:

Where I Need to Plant Healthy Snacks	What Snacks I Will Store There	When and How I Will Do So
My desk drawer at work	Raw almonds	Add an extra bag of nuts to my weekly shopping list every Sunday and bring them in every Monday morning
My carry-on bag when I travel	Salmon jerky, whole-food protein bars (with ingredients like nuts, seeds, and dried fruit), wild dried blueberries	Pin a note to the inside of my carry-on bag so I remember to pack snacks
Around the house on weekends	Crudités and dip in the fridge	Make a batch of dip and cut up vegetables early Saturday mornings, after my morning walk

■ **Steer clear of your danger zones**. If the drive-through you pass each morning on your way to work calls out to you like a siren song, chart another daily route. If the aroma from the bakery you walk past on your way to work is irresistible to you, walk down a different block. Put yourself—literally—on a path to health rather than temptation! Record in your Detox Journal your top danger zones and create a chart like this one:

My Danger Zone	How I Will Avoid It	When I Will Implement My New Plan
The vending machines in the copy room at work	Make my copies on the floor below, where they have no vending machines	Next time I need to use the copy machine

(Continued)

My Danger Zone	How I Will Avoid It	When I Will Implement My New Plan
The concession stand at the field where my child plays soccer	Set up my chair on the opposite side of the field, away from the concession stand, and bring my own drinks and snacks so I am not tempted	This Saturday

■ **Protect your health bubble in social situations.** When and with whom do you find yourself feeling pressured or tempted to eat or drink things that work against your health goals? At work when they bring in platters of food and soda for lunch? When you are out with friends? At holidays with family? Identify your top three temptation zones (ideally ones that are current or immediately upcoming) and write in your Detox Journal your specific plan to protect yourself in those situations. Strategies include bringing your own food to events, telling your family about your eating plan so they are on board and supportive of your efforts, or eating some raw veggies and dip before you go out to dinner with friends so you are not so hungry and at the mercy of the bread basket. Your chart might look something like this:

My Temptation Zone	My Strategy	How/When I Will Make It Happen
Dinner parties	Offer to bring one healthy dish I will eat	In three weeks, when we are going to the Smiths' house for dinner

My Temptation Zone	My Strategy	How/When I Will Make It Happen
Out to dinner with my family	Ask my family to support me in my weight loss efforts (and respect my decision not to share desserts with them). Or pick the restaurant myself and find one with healthy options	This Friday night
Friday lunch meetings at work	Bring my own lunch so I am not tempted by the platters	Prepare lunch in advance every Thursday night

■ **Make exercise easy.** Identify the top three obstacles that get in the way of your daily exercise. Is it having the clothing you need, clean and easy to access? When the weather is bad? Make a backup plan for your daily walk if the weather is bad (use the treadmill at a gym, try a workout DVD, etc.). Think about systems you can put into place to trigger you to do the right thing. For example, I hate push-ups, but I like showers, so every day before I get in the shower I do thirty to forty push-ups (I could only do ten when I started!). Write your specific plan in your Detox Journal for making exercise automatic and enjoyable. Other examples include:

My Exercise Obstacle	My Strategy	How/When I Will Make It Happen
Inclement weather	Use the treadmill at the gym	Next rainy day
Lack of time	Build a thirty-minute exercise routine into my daily schedule as a permanent commitment	Input this into my electronic calendar so the time is automatically blocked off. (use the seven-minute workout at the end of Day 4 as a back up.

(Continued)

My Exercise Obstacle	My Strategy	How/When I Will Make It Happen
Boredom	Try a new fitness class	Register today for a Pilates class next Tuesday night

▪ **Keep your supplies for self-nurturing practices at the ready.**
What three things can you do to keep your relaxation practices going?
Ideas might include keeping your bathroom cabinet stocked with extra
Epsom salts, baking soda, and lavender oil, so you always have what you
need to take an UltraDetox Bath. Set a timer to remind you to do your
meditation awareness practice. Think about what gives you peace and
triggers your relaxation response, then set up your defaults so you can
do those practices often. Create a chart in your Detox Journal like the
following:

Relaxation Practice I Will Continue	How I Will Make It Easy and Automatic to Do So	When I Will Implement My Plan
Take-Five Breathing Break before every meal	Put a note in my silverware drawer, so when I reach for a utensil to eat I am automatically reminded	Tonight
Meditation practice	Put a daily alert on my phone to go off each evening at 8 p.m.	As soon as I am done with this journal entry
Walking with my best friend on Saturday mornings	Every Friday night, check in with my friend to confirm we are on for the following morning	This Friday night

Assemble Your Emergency Life Pack

If you had a bee-sting allergy or a peanut allergy, you would never leave the house without an EpiPen. Likewise, if you have a body, you need an emergency life pack so you are never stranded without healthy options. It makes sense that if you want to survive our toxic nutritional food environment, you need to make and carry your own survival kit. See www.10daydetox.com/resources for specific brands and where to find the best items for your Emergency Life Pack. Here's what's in mine:

Nonperishable items

Wild canned salmon

Canned sardines

Salmon jerky

Natural turkey jerky or grass- or pasture-raised beef (with no nitrates)

Almonds, walnuts, pumpkin seeds

Nut butters (almond, macadamia nut, walnut)

Coconut butter (in individual packets)

Mary's Gone Crackers gluten-free flaxseed crackers

Jar of artichoke hearts

Whole-food protein bars

Unsweetened dried wild blueberries

Water

Some Perishable Items for a Cooler

Hard-boiled eggs

Hummus (can be found in nonperishable little serving packets)

Carrot and celery sticks, sliced cucumber, cherry tomatoes

Apple or pear

I have emergency food in my car, in my office drawers, and in my travel bag. Have fun creating your own Emergency Life Pack!

16

Day 9: Notice

It had been over a year since my last exam because I didn't want to know the numbers. Well, denial is definitely not a remedy. I decided I wanted to know — needed to know — my starting point so I could track my progress. I wanted to know ALL of the numbers, not just lab results but body measurements, too.

I dove into the detox thinking, "I'll do my part, Dr. Hyman, and let's see just how good things can be in only ten days." After ten days, almost all of my numbers improved. I was amazed! I lost 7 pounds and a total of 11.5 inches from my whole body. My glucose went from 88 to 73, insulin went from 11 to 6, triglycerides from 197 to 140, and my total cholesterol dropped by 64 points.

All of this tracking gave the whole experience a different feel. For the first time I felt like I wasn't trying another "diet." Tracking the numbers gave everything more purpose and helped me become completely engaged in my process. It's as if I'm my own science experiment with guaranteed positive results. The best part? Decreases in clothing size. As a result of the Blood Sugar Solution 10-Day Detox Diet, I went down one whole size. Looking at the numbers in black and white is powerfully affirming and motivating.

How good can things get from here? I don't know yet…I'm still on the journey. At the end of the 10-Day Detox Dr. Hyman challenged us to continue the plan for another ninety days. If things could improve so much in a mere ten days, just imagine what could happen after ninety more!

— ANGELA JANNOTTA

Morning:

- Take your measurements and record your results in your Detox Journal or online tracking tool. Also record how many hours you slept the night before and the quality of that sleep.
- Begin the day with thirty minutes of brisk walking or other exercise.
- Just before breakfast, take 2.5 to 5 grams of PGX fiber: 3 to 6 capsules or ½ to 1 scoop of the powder in 10 ounces of water.
- Take the rest of your supplements (see page 118) with breakfast.
- Make your Breakfast Detox Shake (see menu plan below).
- Optional: Enjoy a midmorning snack (see menu plan below).

Afternoon:

- Just before lunch, take 2.5 to 5 grams of PGX fiber with water.
- Eat lunch (see menu plan below).
- Optional: Enjoy a midafternoon snack (see menu plan below).

Evening:

- Just before dinner, take 2.5 to 5 grams of PGX fiber with a glass of water.
- Take the rest of your supplements (see page 118) with dinner.
- Eat dinner (see menu plan below).
- Spend fifteen minutes recording your experience and answering the Day 9 Journal Questions listed on page 199. Write down everything you ate and did today, how you feel, any improvements or changes in your energy and focus, and how these changes make you feel physically, mentally, and emotionally.
- Practice the Take-Five Breathing Break (see page 121) for 5 minutes.
- Take your twenty-to-thirty-minute UltraDetox Bath (see page 122).
- Get seven to eight hours of sleep.

Today's Meals:

- Breakfast: Detox Shake (page 267)

- Midmorning Snack (optional): 10 to 12 nuts (almonds, walnuts, pecans, macadamia nuts)
- Lunch:
  - Core Plan: Soup with protein (page 273) or Dr. Hyman's Super Salad Bar with protein (page 271)
  - Adventure Plan: Spiced Turkey Wrap with Watercress and Avocado (page 298)
- Midafternoon Snack (optional): Dip or spread of your choice (page 316) with fresh vegetables
- Dinner:
  - Core Plan: Steamed Snapper with Ginger and Scallions (page 286)
  - Adventure Plan: Thai Fish Salad (page 313)

Today's Focus: Notice

Most of us go through life unconscious of how much we eat, how much we sleep, how much we relax, even how much money we spend. But in order to transform your habits, you first need to be aware of what they look like so you know what needs to change. You may be drinking six Diet Cokes a day and not even realizing it!

When I have patients track their diet and blood sugar, blood pressure, weight, waist, and hip size, suddenly they can understand how quickly and dramatically their health can be affected by whatever they eat—even by something as simple as a bowl of cereal.

Not long ago, I spent time with the Abbot of Menri at his Tibetan monastery in northern India. He thought he was eating a good, healthy breakfast every day. It was the traditional Tibetan breakfast called *tsampa,* eaten by yak herders for centuries, which consists of roasted barley with yak cheese and salty tea. There was only one problem: The abbot wasn't herding yaks at 15,000 feet, but rather herding monks into the meditation hall. I convinced him to let his assistant test his blood sugar two hours after eating that meal, and it spiked up to 350 mg/dl (normal is less than 100 mg/dl). At first he blamed the machine, certain it was broken! I assured him it wasn't; to prove it, I checked my blood sugar and that of another monk having breakfast with us, and both were normal. It was one thing for me to tell the abbot that this breakfast wasn't good for him, but another for him to see it with his own eyes. He immediately changed his breakfast to one that would balance his blood sugar. And now his hemoglobin A1c, or average blood sugar, went from over 8.0 to under 6.0 and he lost thirty pounds (thirteen kilos).

Those who track their thoughts, emotions, and experiences have real proof of the changes that are possible. It might seem annoying at the beginning to measure yourself, write down your numbers, track your labs, what you are eating, how much you move and exercise, how much you sleep or relax, but the science shows that this dramatically magnifies your success. Think about it this

> I normally concentrate on what I choose to eat and hadn't realized I had gotten so lax. By tracking what I do every day I gained a deeper understanding of where unhealthy foods creep in and how I can take back control and still be satisfied with the foods I'm eating.
>
> —SHERRY TREBES

way: If you lost twenty pounds (nine kilos) without tracking, you could lose forty pounds (18 kilos) just by measuring and recording your results. The simple act of becoming conscious and noticing shifts behavior and habits.

We only have two more days to go on the program, and I want to give you some lasting strategies for practicing awareness so that you can keep making progress even after you've completed the formal part of this detox plan.

Strategies for Awareness

■ Record the following in your Detox Journal each day (or begin a new Transition Journal once the ten days are over). Be as specific as possible:

Measurements

- Weight
- Hips
- Thighs
- Blood sugar
- Blood pressure

Actions

- What went into your mouth (what foods or drinks, with portion sizes) and how you felt after eating it, both immediately and a few hours later
- How much and what exercise you did, and how you felt afterward
- How many hours of sleep you got and how it affected you the next day
- What relaxation practices you did (breathing exercises, UltraDetox Bath, etc.), and how you felt afterward

Reflection

- What you notice about how you look and feel physically
- What you notice about your moods and emotions
- What you notice about your energy levels
- What you notice about your thoughts (what you're focused on, how your thinking patterns appear to be changing, etc.)

■ **Fill out the Toxicity Questionnaire** on pages 5–7 at the end of the ten days, and again every two weeks to track specific health changes.

■ **Get tech-savvy.** There are a lot of smart new products and apps that are built to help you quantify and track your activity and progress. I encourage you to use these. You can share and compare your results with others and get support for your success and a nudge when you are off track. Some of my favorites are FitBit and Withings Pulse, which wirelessly sync to your computer and smartphone, and UP by Jawbone, a wristband that records your physical activity and hours of sleep and connects to your iPhone for easy tracking of your numbers. The FitBit Aria Wi-Fi Smart Scale or the Withings scale and separate blood pressure cuff automatically sync up data about your weight, body composition, body mass index, and blood pressure with your profile on your computer and smartphone. Online programs such as heartmath.com and quantifiedself.com offer other great ways to stay accountable and also to tap into a like-minded community.

> I can really see the difference in my energy levels and how I feel when I don't eat sugar. I have energy all day and don't have as many headaches. I'm going to make a change in the amount of sugar I put into my body after this.
>
> — SHANNON CREEKMUR

Day 9 Journal Questions

- How do I feel physically?
- What changes do I notice in my body?
- What thoughts and emotions are present for me today?
- How did it feel to track my results and experiences during this program? How did it affect me?
- What surprised me the most about my results and experiences?
- Where, when, and how will I record my results and other things I notice about my body going forward?

Bonus: Take a Look Back

Take a few minutes tonight to read through your journal entries, beginning on Day 1. What do you notice about how you felt then as compared to now? Do you remember feeling the way you did on Day 1? How are you different than you were just nine days ago? Most people are amazed at how far they've come, and you've got your own evolution recorded as proof!

17

Day 10: Connect

Negative lifestyle choices and high job stress led me down a path of alcohol and nicotine abuse, and eventually open heart surgery. After my recovery, I watched myself transfer my addiction from alcohol and cigarettes to food. I quickly gained thirty pounds and heightened my carb and sugar cravings. I knew I was headed for more problems as my blood sugar continued to rise and I started experiencing blurred vision, muscle aches and pains, dizziness, and more. My doctor started me on insulin shots. I spent many hours reading everything I could get my hands on about diet and nutrition. I continued to eat and read, read and eat. Apparently, the urgency to act still eluded me.

When my sister e-mailed telling me about the 10-Day Detox trial program she had signed up for, I knew it was time. I would not be around much longer if I continued to punish myself with damaging dietary habits. I had the knowledge required…I just needed the structure and support to get me started. My sister lives in Fort Worth and I live in Houston, so I drove up and stayed with her so we could experience and support each other through the program.

Together, she and I learned that the typical American "comfort food" didn't give us comfort in the long run. We learned together how to start cooking with spices and alternative plant-based fats. We never felt deprived, and as a result, felt satisfied and encouraged. My blood sugar started at 369, and today, twelve days later, I am down to 156 with no insulin. One reading even got down to 138! I have lost ten pounds, my BMI went from 31.9 to 30.1, and I have lost 1.75 inches in my waist. Our plan together is to continue for another ninety days and see where it leads us.

— KAREN SHELTON

Morning:

- Take your measurements and record your results in your Detox Journal or online tracking tool. Also record how many hours you slept the night before and the quality of that sleep.
- Begin the day with thirty minutes of brisk walking or other exercise.
- Just before breakfast, take 2.5 to 5 grams of PGX fiber: 3 to 6 capsules or ½ to 1 scoop of the powder in 10 ounces of water.
- Take the rest of your supplements with breakfast.
- Make your Breakfast Detox Shake (see menu plan below).
- Optional: Enjoy a midmorning snack (see menu plan below).

Afternoon:

- Just before lunch, take 2.5 to 5 grams of PGX fiber with water.
- Eat lunch (see menu plan below).
- Optional: Enjoy a midafternoon snack (see menu plan below).

Evening:

- Just before dinner, take 2.5 to 5 grams of PGX fiber with water.
- Take the rest of your supplements (see page 118) with dinner.
- Eat dinner (see menu plan below).
- Spend fifteen minutes recording your experience and answering the Day 10 Journal Questions listed on page 206. Write down everything you ate and did today, how you feel, any improvements or changes in your energy and focus, and how these changes make you feel physically, mentally, and emotionally.
- Do the Take-Five Breathing Break (see page 121).
- Take your twenty-to-thirty-minute UltraDetox Bath (see page 122).
- Get seven to eight hours of sleep.

Today's Meals:

- Breakfast: Detox Shake (page 267)

- Midmorning Snack (optional): 10 to 12 nuts (almonds, walnuts, pecans, macadamia nuts)
- Lunch:
  - Core Plan: Soup with protein (page 273) or Dr. Hyman's Super Salad Bar with protein (page 271)
  - Adventure Plan: Watercress and Arugula Salad with Poached Eggs (page 299)
- Midafternoon Snack (optional): Dip or spread of your choice (page 316) with fresh vegetables
- Dinner:
  - Core Plan: Grilled Tofu with Cilantro Pesto (page 286)
  - Adventure Plan: Chicken Encrusted with Red Chili Pesto (page 315)

Today's Focus: Connect

Congratulations—you made it! After today you will have completed the 10-Day Detox. I hope you are feeling vibrant, healthy, and best of all, proud of what you've accomplished!

The short-term goals you've achieved over these ten days can be life-changing—if you take the steps to make sure they stick. Now more than ever, as you enter the transition phase, it's crucial to harness the power of community for your continued success. Hopefully, you have found a buddy, or a partner, or even created or joined a group to support you on your journey to vibrant good health and weight loss. Or perhaps you joined the Blood Sugar Solution 10-Day Detox Diet Online Course and connected with the online community or a small group at www.10daydetox.com/resources.

If you have, that's fabulous. I encourage you to stay connected, to meet weekly, to touch base and check in about how you feel and what you need to support long-term success. If not, consider making it a priority now. Remember that in our Daniel Plan study, those who did the program together lost twice as much weight as those who did it alone, even though they were all otherwise following the *same* program. Life is full of challenges, and finding (or creating) your community is a powerful way to manage, process, and thrive through all the ups and downs. We need the support of others to make lasting shifts in how we eat, move, and live. We're better together—it's as simple as that.

You probably have loved ones in your life whose support you want in your continuing journey. Even though these people may care deeply for you, they may not know how to support you in your health and weight loss efforts. It's your job to teach them. Here are some strategies to help your loved ones get on board as part of your continuing support team:

■ **Share your plan.** Explain what your dream is and your plan for achieving that dream, and ask those near you for the specific help you need. For example, you may tell your best friends that your dream is to be living in a healthy and toned body by summertime, and your plan is to follow the Blood Sugar Solution 10-Day Detox Diet transition plan. You can then ask your friends to remember that this plan means no alcohol or sugary munchies when you eat out with them, and to remind you of your plan if you seem to be caving in to your cravings.

■ **Deal with feedback.** If others are not on the same journey you are, they may not understand it. That is normal. Some people may question what you are doing, saying things like "But you seem perfectly healthy to me" or "That way of eating just isn't normal." Remember that comments like these are usually well-intentioned attempts to make you feel good about yourself as you are. See the care behind these comments, but don't use them as an excuse to veer off your eating plan. Thank your friends for their concern, explain why you are on the plan, and ask them directly and specifically for the support you need. This may mean asking them kindly not to tell you that you are "fine as is," because you are striving for a greater level of wellness, or telling them that their support would mean a lot to you, even if they don't quite get why you are doing this.

■ **Convey the attitude you want reflected back at you.** The world is a mirror. For your loved ones to celebrate your eating plan, *you* need to celebrate your eating plan. If you have the attitude of "Ugh, this diet is so hard. It's killing me. Only two more days left of this torture!", then the people around you will pick up on that and mirror it by saying things like "Take it easy, this program is nuts, I think you should stop it." Whereas if you express the empowered and energetic attitude of "This detox program is amazing. Yes, it's hard at times, but it's so worth it and I am so proud of myself for doing it," then the people in your life will mirror this back and be happy for you.

Not only is it important to gather the support of your loved ones as you embark on your journey to health, but it's also important for you to build a network of community support that will accompany you on that journey. This community will help you stick to your new health habits and hold you accountable for following them. Below you'll find some strategies for building a health-supporting community.

Strategies for Connecting

▪ **Join the 10-Day Detox Diet online community or course** at www.10daydetox.com/resources if you haven't already. There you will find others who are doing the detox and transitioning to the next phase, as you are about to do. You can share your experience, swap ideas and tips, and receive support and encouragement. Being part of a group of like-minded folks with a common purpose such as this can mean the difference between success and failure. We are social beings. Chronic illness, especially obesity and diabetes, is a social disease and needs a social cure. **The group is the medicine; the community is the cure.** This is the most powerful part of the 10-Day Detox program, and essential for long-term success.

▪ **Start the Daniel Plan** at your church, temple, synagogue, mosque, or other community center (go to www.danielplan.com for more info).

▪ **Start a lunch club at work** and take turns bringing in healthy lunches for the group. That way you only have to cook once every week or two.

■ **Form a supper club** with your neighbors or friends once a week or once a month to connect with and support one another. Make it an event. Shop and/or cook and eat together. Pick a topic to engage everyone in a discussion of meaning: food, relationships, self-care, or anything that is authentic, real, and connecting.

■ **Choose one "health buddy"** in your life to team up and check in with every day, or at least once a week. Report in on what you've been eating, exercise you've had, changes you notice in your body, how you feel. Cheer each other on and lend support when one of you hits a roadblock.

■ **Inspire your friends and family by becoming a 10-Day Detox Group Leader.** After you've finished your ten days, find six to ten people who want to do the detox and lead your own Blood Sugar Solution 10-Day Detox group. You can get a complete guide on how to lead a group at www.10daydetox.com/resources, or join the Blood Sugar Solution 10-Day Detox Diet Online Course to get daily support and encouragement from me and my nutrition coaches and join an online group at www.10daydetox.com/resources.

■ **Join a fitness club, sports team, or other physical activity club.** This is a great way to connect with people who enjoy the same things you do. Like to run? Check out your local running club. If yoga is your thing, find a studio you love and go to it regularly—yoga people are very friendly, and you'll find companions in no time. Sign up to play in a basketball league...even bowling...Whatever you love to do, find a group and become a part of it.

Day 10 is here. At first I wasn't sure I could make it for ten days, but this has been so easy! I will continue to nourish my body in this wonderful way because I feel so good now. I have more energy and I feel that I am thinking more clearly than I have in a long, long time. Real and natural foods are in my future.

— ROBERTA PRESSLER

Day 10 Journal Questions

- How do I feel physically?
- What thoughts and emotions are present for me today?
- What changes in my body do I notice?
- With whom might I form a support group?
- Where in my life, or at the periphery of my life, do healthy communities exist?
- Where in my life might there be a latent community waiting for me to mobilize it?
- What keeps me from reaching out to others for support and connection?
- How has my experience in going through this program been enhanced by community?
- What are my plans for creating connection and community going forward to support my health and weight loss success?

THE GREATEST GIFT

The gift of ten days dedicated to yourself is like no other you can ever give or receive. Yes, you detoxed from sugar and junk and addictive habits. But you also gave yourself the chance to connect with yourself— to examine your thoughts and beliefs, and the ways in which you live that don't support the greatest expression of who you are. Ten days may not seem like a lot, but I hope it gave you a taste of what is possible.

The reason I created this program was to give you a profound experience of how quickly you can feel better, to show you how health, energy, weight loss, and, yes, even happiness are available to you when you use food as medicine and make a few simple changes in your day. Once you have experienced what it feels like to feel good, to get rid of brain fog, cravings, joint pain, fatigue, excess weight, and a myriad of other chronic health problems, then you know there is a path forward. I encourage you to see this as the first step on a new path of caring for yourself, of eating and living in a way that helps you thrive for the rest of your life.

You now have the knowledge and skills you need to recharge your life, and this program can be a touchstone that you can return to whenever you need to reset. I still need it, just like everyone else. In fact, I do this program myself four times a year—not to lose weight, but to reboot my life. It's like a vacation without going anywhere. For me it's a form of self-created paradise. I hope it is for you, too!

PART V

THE TRANSITION PHASE

18

After the Detox

I feel like my body has just come out of the dentist office after a cleaning. You know that feeling of never wanting to eat or drink anything to disturb that sense of CLEAN? Well, the clean is now on the whole inside, and I don't want to lose this feeling! The meals were and will be a special gift that I will be giving myself, hopefully every day of my life. Actually, now there is no choice. Even my dog is trimming down from eating healthy treats!

— ANGELA PEZZA

Congratulations! You have completed what I hope are the first ten days of an entirely new way of living—an introduction to a much higher level of wellness and sense of control over your food choices. This program is really my sneaky way of getting you to see for yourself how little is truly separating you from health and happiness. It's really not complicated! Your body is a biological organism, and you only have to understand its basic operation to get it to function optimally. You now have the experiential knowledge of how to create health and lose weight safely and easily, and that kind of wisdom is priceless.

So what now?

This program has given you a small taste of what is possible, and now it's up to you to decide the path you want to follow to take your health and weight loss to even greater levels. In this chapter, I'm going to give you three different transitional paths you can choose from: the Super Advanced Plan, the Advanced Plan, and the Basic Plan. Each of these is designed for specific goals, but all are guaranteed to keep the success going. After that, I'll give you the Blood Sugar Solution for Life, your template for staying slim and healthy forever.

But first, before you head into your transition, it's good to do a little mental debriefing and take some final tests and measurements. This will help you to preserve what's fresh in your mind about your experience, as well as to see the full scope of your results.

YOUR PERSONAL "EXIT INTERVIEW"

Right now, you are in a great, clear space in both mind and body. I want you to capture that clarity in writing as a reminder of what's possible, and what you—and your body—are capable of. I encourage you not to skip over this valuable step. You have gained a wealth of insight and knowledge through your ten-day experience. Now's the time to commit your key takeaways to paper so you can come back to them whenever you need fresh inspiration and motivation.

Open to a blank page in your Detox Journal and clear some time to write your answers to the following questions:

- What have I learned about my body over the past ten days?
- What did I notice or discover about my relationship to food?
- What did I notice about my energy levels?
- What did I notice about how my sleep (amount and quality) affected me the following day?
- How did I effectively handle difficult or challenging moments?
- Which practices did I enjoy the most, and why?
- Which practices do I want to continue, and how will I implement that?
- What benefits did I get from the community support?
- What do I want for myself going forward?

That final question is all about looking ahead. With a vision of your chosen future and goals clearly in mind, you can decide which of the following transition plans is right for you.

RETAKE THE TOXICITY QUESTIONNAIRE

> In the past year I found out I have a thyroid problem. I gained thirty-five pounds and had not been able to lose any weight, and I am so tired all the time. The doctor kept upping my medicine and at 125 micrograms of Synthroid I felt no different. Then this program came along. What a difference the last ten days have made in my life! I have hope again. I lost weight and feel terrific. I finally feel my thyroid is responding to something. I will continue on with your advice forever. Also, my cravings are a thing of the past...I can actually walk down the dessert aisle now and keep walking.
>
> — PAULETTA DOUGHTY

Now that you are at the end of your ten days, I encourage you to go back and complete the "after" section in the Toxicity Questionnaire on pages 5–7. I think you're going to be amazed by the changes! During the Blood Sugar Solution 10-Day Detox trial program, one of the most extraordinary outcomes was seeing participants' average toxicity score go down by 42 points (62 percent). That is the power of food, and the power of the body to recover and heal.

WHAT IF YOU DIDN'T LOSE WEIGHT OR FEEL BETTER?

There are a few people (a very small minority) who, despite having done their best to follow this program, may still not feel that much better or lose that much weight. This is a clue that there is something else going on. Don't be discouraged—there is a solution! These are findable, fixable problems if you know where to look.

If you completed the 10-Day Detox and did not get the results you were hoping for, one of the following five reasons might apply:

1. **Problems with diet.** Did sugar or gluten sneak its way into your food products? Your success can easily be sabotaged by hidden sources.

Check your labels carefully—or better yet, eat only fresh foods without labels.

2. **Inadequate or inefficient exercise.** If you have never exercised, a little exercise can create large benefits at first. However, as you progress and get healthier, you need higher-intensity workouts to achieve the same benefits. As you get into shape, increase your exercise and intensity and add in interval training (see pages 154–55 for more on this).

3. **Hidden food sensitivities.** Some people have food allergies or sensitivities (besides gluten or dairy) that can prevent weight loss. This calls for a more comprehensive elimination diet. In my book *The Ultra-Simple Diet* you can find a powerful, healing anti–inflammatory elimination program to help you identify the degree to which food sensitivities or allergies may be driving the inflammation. Other common allergens include eggs, corn, soy, nuts, nightshades (the tomato, potato, eggplant, and pepper family), yeast, and citrus foods. You may also need food-sensitivity testing, which you can learn more about in my free online guide, *How to Work with Your Doctor to Get What You Need,* at www.10daydetox.com/resources.

4. **Toxic overload.** Accumulation of toxins from substances such as petrochemicals and heavy metals can cause problems in many people who are overexposed to them or who have genetic predispositions that make it difficult to detoxify these chemicals. If this is a problem for you, you might need heavy-metal detoxification protocols, saunas, and various detoxifying supplements, including n-acetyl-cysteine, milk thistle, and vitamin C. For more information, please see Chapter 24 of *The Blood Sugar Solution.* (Note: Heavy-metal detoxification is a medical procedure that requires the guidance of an experienced functional medicine doctor. See *How to Work with Your Doctor to Get What You Need* at www.10daydetox.com/resources for more information on finding the right doctor for testing and detoxing for heavy metals.)

5. **Systemic imbalances.** In functional medicine, we see the body as a system. The root causes of disease trigger imbalances in the body that lead to dysfunction. Many things can go wrong that affect your

health. Here are the main triggers that interact with your genes to cause most disease: toxins, allergens, microbes, stress, and poor diet. These can cause nutritional deficiencies, hormonal imbalances (including thyroid and adrenal and sex-hormone problems), imbalances in your gut flora or microbiome, immune imbalances, inflammation from hidden infections, problems with energy metabolism, and more. These imbalances often require attention from a well-trained functional medicine doctor (read below for more on how to find one).

Unfortunately, most doctors today are not trained to find toxic overload or systemic imbalances, or to treat them effectively. My guide *How to Work with Your Doctor to Get What You Need* outlines how to identify all these problems and more, what tests to have, and what treatments are available; it even gives you a template for a letter explaining to your doctor why he or she should help you be a detective. You are welcome to come see one of the doctors at my clinic in Massachusetts, the Ultra-Wellness Center, or find a functional medicine doctor close to you by going to www.functionalmedicine.org and entering your zip code in the "find a practitioner" section.

Please keep in mind that not all the health professionals in the database are equally skilled or trained, so you'll want to make some additional inquiries before selecting a practitioner. Ask the candidates you are considering if they have gone through the Functional Medicine Certification Program, which represents a higher level of training.

Thankfully, there is a road to health for almost everyone, given the right guidance and support. Sometimes it takes a bit of detective work, with hidden clues that need sorting out. If you work with a well-trained functional medicine practitioner, you can reclaim your health.

RECHECK YOUR LAB TESTS

If you did basic lab tests before beginning the 10-Day Detox, I encourage you to repeat the same tests six weeks from the day you started the detox. If you stick with one of the Blood Sugar Solution 10-Day Detox Diet transition plans, you will be amazed by the changes. Some may see drops of fifty or more points in their blood sugar or cholesterol after just ten days, but after one month, you will be shocked by the even more dramatic changes. Seeing these numbers change will go a long way in reinforcing your commitment to yourself.

YOUR CONTINUING JOURNEY

Whichever transition plan you choose, it is my hope that you will continue with some of the practices you have adopted over these past ten days. It's not magic that made your cravings disappear, your energy sky-

> How many programs end and you still want to do them? My whole attitude is so good, my energy level is up, and I feel so much better. This is a spectacular feat for a ten-day period.
> — JUDY KNIGHT

rocket, your skin clear up, your digestion improve, your joints and muscles stop hurting, your headaches go away, or your brain fog clear up. It is no accident that you look and feel as fabulous as you do. *You* made this happen!

The eating plans, UltraDetox Baths, breathing exercises, results tracking, journaling, daily exercise, community support, conscious design of your "health bubble"...these are all powerful ways to keep your body and mind steered in the direction of health and sustainable weight loss. You've regained control of your body and your life, and there's no going back!

THE SUPER ADVANCED PLAN

> I'm in for another ninety days. I lost six pounds and three inches off my waist and belly. Can't beat that! My blood sugar has dropped to normal and I can't wait for my next doctor visit to see how my blood panels look.

My family history is full of diabetes. Both of my grandmothers had it… both of my brothers have it…my dad and mom are both pre-diabetic, and I was headed in that direction. But I am CHOOSING a different path. Congratulations to everyone here who has also started choosing a better, healthier future for themselves and their families!

— TERRI GARVIN

The Super Advanced Plan is the same plan you followed during the 10-Day Detox. When I launched the trial of the 10-Day Detox, I challenged the participants to continue for an additional ninety days so they could reach even higher levels of health and weight loss. Many of them were up for the challenge, and after the first six weeks the results continued to amaze both them and me:

- Participants experienced an average weight loss of 8.1 (3.5 kg) pounds in the first ten days and an average loss of 14 (6.5 kg) pounds over the following six weeks (some people reached their healthiest weight and didn't need to lose any more, thus they didn't, while others lost a lot more than 14 pounds/6.5 kg).
- Their waist size went down by an average of 1.7 inches in the first ten days, and 3.2 inches over six weeks.
- Their hip size went down 1.5 inches in the first ten days and 2.7 inches over six weeks.
- The average blood pressure dropped ten points after six weeks.
- The average blood sugar dropped about eighteen points after six weeks.

Follow the Super Advanced Plan if you:

- Want to lose twenty-five pounds (eleven kilos) or more.
- Have diabetes and want to reverse it.

- Are on diabetes medication or insulin and want to get off it.
- Have high triglycerides and low HDL (good cholesterol) and want to get off statin medication.
- Have high blood pressure and want to get off medication.
- Just feel so great and want to keep going to experience greater levels of wellness.

Here is the protocol for the Super Advanced Plan:

- Follow the same daily guidelines as laid out in Chapter 7, "Your Daily Practices."
- Continue to eliminate all gluten and flour-based products (including gluten-free), dairy, and all forms of sugar and sweeteners.
- Continue to avoid all processed foods.
- Avoid grains, starchy vegetables (like potatoes), beans, and fruit (other than ½ cup of berries or kiwi in your morning shake).
- Avoid inflammatory beverages (regular and decaf coffee, alcohol, soda, and juice).
- Include as many nonstarchy vegetables as you want in all meals and snacks.
- Include 4 to 6 ounces of protein with each meal (eggs, chicken, fish, lean animal protein, nuts and seeds).
- Have one serving of a healthy fat (e.g., ¼ avocado, or 1 tablespoon extra virgin olive oil, walnut oil, sesame oil, extra virgin coconut butter, or nut or seed butter such as almond or cashew) with every meal.
- Continue with your daily practices: thirty minutes of exercise, supplements, Take-Five Breathing Break, UltraDetox Bath, journaling, tracking results, hydration, and seven to eight hours sleep every night.
- Continue to take the same supplements that you have been taking during the 10-Day Detox. Additionally, you'll need to add a few more nutrients and herbs to further stabilize your blood sugar balance and improve insulin sensitivity. These herbs are often available as combinations. I've listed the dosages below, or you can order the

10-Day Detox Step-Up Pack, which includes all of these, at www.10daydetox.com/resources (or you can order both the 10-Day Detox Supplement Pack and the 10-Day Detox Step-Up Pack combined in one package; this is called the 10-Day Detox Combo Pack).

- 600 milligrams alpha lipoic acid twice a day
- 1,000 milligrams fenugreek seed with each meal
- 150 milligrams bitter melon with each meal
- 100 milligrams gymnema leaf with each meal
- 540 milligrams acacia bark extract (iso-alpha acids) once daily

You can continue to use your favorite recipes from *The Blood Sugar Solution 10-Day Detox Diet,* and you might want to try some new ones from *The Blood Sugar Solution Cookbook.* Just be sure to avoid any recipes that contain beans, grains, or starchy vegetables while on the Super Advanced Plan.

What Do I Do if I Veer Off Course?

At some point during your detox experience, you may find yourself thrown off your plan by unanticipated circumstances, distractions, or stresses. If so, just be gentle with yourself. Acknowledge whatever happened and return to the 10-Day Detox Diet without judgment, shame, or blame. Think of it like the soothing voice on your GPS that, when you take a wrong turn, kindly says, "Make your next possible U-turn." Just come back to the tools you've discovered here.

I recommend doing the full 10-Day Detox program again to hit the big reset and get yourself back on track. Now that you have experienced this once, you know that you are only a few days away from wellness and happiness! It is available to you anytime. You have learned the skills; you now have a permanent road map that is yours to keep. If you are human, you will get lost or go off track from time to time. Now you know the way home.

THE ADVANCED PLAN

> My weight went from 176 to 167 during the ten days, and I intend to keep this going. I'll evaluate every thirty days for the next three months, to determine when to move into the next phase. At that point I'll start adding in small amounts of starchy veggies. But no matter what, I will keep this good feeling going, hopefully for the rest of my life. Constant awareness, making it a habit, and putting this into practice every day will keep me on the road to success.
>
> — KATHY THOMPSON

The Advanced Plan is similar to the Super Advanced Plan, except you can now add in legumes (beans and lentils). This is the same Advanced Plan I outlined in my book *The Blood Sugar Solution*.

Follow this plan if you:

- Want to continue to get the benefits of the 10-Day Detox and add beans back to your diet to see how you respond to them (some people with diabesity can't tolerate beans because they contain enough starch to spike blood sugar as well as lectins that create inflammation and weight gain).
- Have advanced diabesity (based on the comprehensive diabesity questionnaire that you can find in *The Blood Sugar Solution* or at www.10daydetox.com/resources). You can also learn more about diabesity and how to stay healthy in the long term by reading *The Blood Sugar Solution*.

Here is the protocol for the Advanced Plan:

- Follow the same daily guidelines as laid out in Chapter 7, "Your Daily Practices."
- Continue to eliminate all gluten and flour–based products (including gluten-free), dairy, and all forms of sugar and sweeteners.

- Continue to avoid processed foods.
- Avoid grains, starchy vegetables, and fruit (other than ½ cup of berries or kiwi in your morning shake).
- Avoid inflammatory beverages (regular and decaf coffee, alcohol, soda, and juice).
- Include as many nonstarchy vegetables as you want in all meals and snacks.
- Include 4 to 6 ounces of protein (eggs, fish, chicken, lean animal protein) or ½ cup beans or legumes per meal (see next page for more on beans).
- Have one serving of a healthy fat (e.g., ¼ avocado or 1 tablespoon extra virgin olive oil, walnut oil, sesame oil, extra virgin coconut butter, or nut or seed butter such as almond or cashew) with every meal.
- Continue with your daily practices: thirty minutes of exercise, supplements (the same ones as on the 10-Day Detox), Take-Five Breathing Break, UltraDetox Bath, journaling, tracking results, hydration, and seven to eight hours sleep.
- Use your favorite recipes from the 10-Day Detox or experiment with some new ones from the "Advanced Plan" section of *The Blood Sugar Solution Cookbook*.
- Continue to take the same supplements that you have been taking during the 10-Day Detox. Additionally, you'll need to add a few more nutrients and herbs to further stabilize your blood sugar balance and improve insulin sensitivity. These herbs are often available together as combinations. I've listed the dosages below, or you can order the 10-Day Detox Step-Up Pack, which includes all of these, at www.10daydetox.com/resources (or you can order both the 10-Day Detox Supplement Pack and the 10-Day Detox Step-Up Pack combined in one package; this is called the 10-Day Detox Combo Pack).
  - 600 milligrams alpha lipoic acid twice a day
  - 1,000 milligrams fenugreek seed with each meal
  - 150 milligrams bitter melon with each meal
  - 100 milligrams gymnema leaf with each meal
  - 540 milligrams acacia bark extract (iso-alpha acids) once daily

> ### *Give Beans a Boost*
>
> The best way to eat legumes is by pairing them with a high-quality protein such as fish or chicken. For example, enjoy 3 ounces of broiled wild salmon served over ⅓ cup of lentils, alongside a plate of lightly sautéed kale for a power lunch or quick dinner.

THE BASIC PLAN

The Basic Plan transitions you into nongluten grains, low-glycemic fruit, and a small amount of starchy vegetables. This plan is the same as the Basic Plan outlined in *The Blood Sugar Solution* and is ideal to keep your healing and weight loss going long-term.

Follow the Basic Plan if:

- You have normal blood sugars and blood pressure but still want to continue with weight loss or still have belly fat.
- You have any health conditions, inflammation, or generally don't feel fabulous.
- You don't have a history of heart disease or diabetes.
- Your lab tests show you are a "skinny fat" person with high triglycerides, low HDL, small LDL particles, high blood sugar and insulin.

Here is the protocol for the Basic Plan:

- Continue to eliminate all gluten and flour-based products (including gluten-free goods), plus dairy, and all forms of sugar and sweeteners.
- Avoid inflammatory beverages (regular and decaf coffee, alcohol, soda, and juice).
- Continue to avoid processed foods.
- Include as many nonstarchy vegetables as you want in all meals and snacks.
- Include 4 to 6 ounces of lean protein in each meal.

- Include gluten-free grains (such as quinoa, black rice, and buckwheat) in their whole-kernel form. Ideally, stick with just one serving per day, but you can occasionally have up to two (see box below for portion sizes). Avoid processed grains or any flour products!
- Include nutrient-dense starchy vegetables such as sweet potatoes and winter squash, ideally just one serving per day, but you can have up to two (see box below for portion sizes).
- Include low-glycemic fruit such as apples, pears, berries, or pomegranate, 1 to 2 servings per day (see box below for portion sizes).
- Include beans and legumes, 1 to 2 servings per day (see box below for portion sizes).
- Have one serving of a healthy fat (e.g., ¼ avocado or 1 tablespoon extra virgin olive oil, walnut oil, sesame oil, extra virgin coconut butter, or nut or seed butter such as almond or cashew) with each meal.
- Continue with your daily practices: thirty minutes of physical exercise, Take-Five Breathing Breaks, UltraDetox Bath, journaling, tracking results, hydration, and seven to eight hours sleep.
- Continue with the 10-Day Detox Basic Supplement Pack, outlined on pages 101–2.
- Use your favorite recipes from the 10-Day Detox or experiment with some new ones from the "Basic Plan" section of *The Blood Sugar Solution Cookbook*.

Portion Sizes for One Serving

- Fruit: 1 medium piece, ½ cup berries, ½ cup mixed fresh fruit, ¼ cup dried fruit (avoid, high in sugar)
- Starchy vegetables: 1 cup winter squash, ½ sweet potato
- Protein: 4 to 6 ounces
- Whole grains: ⅓ cup cooked
- Beans: ⅓ cup cooked or canned
- Nuts or seeds: ¼ cup or one small handful

THE BLOOD SUGAR SOLUTION PLAN FOR LIFE

This is a wonderful way to live your life. The combination of healthy, tasty, satisfying food along with daily exercise and learning to center and relax myself, journaling, and hot baths has been powerful to me. I look forward to continuing this with my boyfriend and to being an example to my kids and friends of how easy and rewarding this way of living is. I look forward to "paying this experience forward"!

— ROBIN SEELEY

The final transition option is the one I recommend choosing after you have cycled through a six-week period or more on any of the above three plans. The Blood Sugar Solution Plan for Life follows the same protocol as the Basic Plan, but it reintroduces gluten and dairy (for those who can tolerate them), as well as the occasional treat. This is indeed a plan meant for life; it proves that health and weight management are easy, doable, and most of all, enjoyable.

Here is the protocol for the Blood Sugar Solution Plan for Life:

- Stay away from liquid sugar calories such as soda or juices, unless you are making fresh-squeezed green vegetable juices, which are fabulous.
- Continue to eliminate all artificial sweeteners.
- Minimize all forms of sugar, but especially avoid foods with added sugars. You can always add a little bit of sugar, maple syrup, or honey to the food you cook yourself. That way you know exactly how much you are getting. Note that you should watch to see if any sweetener (sugar, maple syrup, honey, etc.) triggers an addictive pattern of eating. If so, like some alcoholics or addicts, you may have zero tolerance; I'd encourage you to stay away from any type of sugar or sweetener and get your "sugar" exclusively from whole fresh fruit.

- Minimize inflammatory beverages (regular and decaf coffee and alcohol). One cup of coffee and one glass of wine or alcohol three to four times a week can eventually be well tolerated by most people. Just pay attention and notice how they make you feel.
- Continue to avoid processed foods.
- Include as many nonstarchy vegetables as you want in all meals or snacks. Get in the habit of filling 50 to 75 percent of your plate with nonstarchy veggies (see box on page 255 for a full list of unlimited nonstarchy vegetables).
- Include 4 to 6 ounces of lean protein in each meal.
- Include gluten-free grains in their whole-kernel form: quinoa; black, brown, or red rice; buckwheats; 1 to 2 servings per day (see page 223 for portion sizes).
- Avoid all processed grains or flours (with the exception of the pasta you will use to test gluten according to the instructions on page 228).
- Include nutrient-dense starchy vegetables such as sweet potatoes and winter squash, up to 2 servings per day (see page 223 for portion sizes).
- Include low-glycemic fruit such as apples, pears, berries, or pomegranate, 1 to 2 servings per day (see page 223 for portion sizes).
- Include a moderate amount of beans and legumes, 1 to 2 servings per day (see page 223 for portion sizes).
- Have one serving of a healthy fat (e.g., ¼ avocado or 1 tablespoon extra virgin olive oil, walnut oil, or sesame oil, extra virgin coconut butter, or nut or seed butter such as almond or cashew) with each meal.
- Continue with your daily practices: thirty minutes of physical exercise, Take-Five Breathing Breaks, UltraDetox Bath, journaling, tracking results, hydration, and seven to eight hours sleep.
- Continue with the 10-Day Detox Basic Supplement Pack, outlined on pages 101–2.
- Use your favorite recipes from the 10-Day Detox or experiment with some new ones from the "Basic Plan" section of *The Blood Sugar Solution Cookbook*.

- Reintroduce gluten and dairy by following the steps detailed below.

Note: If you are trying to get healthier, lose more weight, or get better control of your blood sugar, stick to one serving (not two) of the beans, grains, or starchy vegetables.

How do I manage when I go out to restaurants?

Eating out should be fun and enjoyable. Choose restaurants in your area that serve real food and that can support your needs and accommodate your requests. Don't be afraid to ask for what you want (whatever it takes to protect your personal "health bubble"). I do it all the time, and so can you! Most good restaurants will take requests to serve simple foods. After all, if you had a life-threatening peanut allergy or shellfish allergy, they wouldn't cook your food in peanut oil or serve you shrimp.

Here are some of my favorite tips for dining out and staying healthy:

- **Be selective.** Choose the restaurant, if possible, when dining with others.
- **Be obnoxious!** Be clear about your needs and do not accept any food that does not nourish or support you. Do not assume you are being impolite; you are simply taking care of yourself.
- **Tell the server you do not want bread on the table, nor the alcoholic beverage menu.** But do ask for raw cut-up veggies without dip.
- **Ask for water.** Drink one or two glasses before your meal to reduce your appetite.
- **Tell the server you will die if you have gluten or dairy.** It's not really a lie — you're just talking about a slow death.
- **Ask for simple food preparation.** Order grilled fish with a plate of steamed vegetables drizzled with olive oil and lemon. Always ask for extra virgin olive oil and lemon in lieu of dressing.
- **Skip the starches.** Ask for double vegetables. Or order an extra side or two of veggies.

- **Avoid sauces, dressings, and dips.** They are usually laden with hidden sugars, unhealthy oils, gluten, and dairy.
- **Always combine carbohydrates (except nonstarchy veggies) with some fiber, protein, or anti-inflammatory fats** (such as extra virgin olive oil, avocado, coconut butter, or nuts) to mitigate blood sugar spikes. Never carb it alone!
- **Focus on protein.** Choosing your protein first is really helpful to ensure that your blood sugar will be balanced and you will eat the right portion size.
- **Ask for berries for dessert.** These are fine to eat alone as long as you have had some protein, fiber, or anti-inflammatory fats within the same meal.

For more tips and ideas, download my free *Restaurant Rescue Guide* at www.10daydetox.com/resources.

Reintroducing Gluten and Dairy

The process for reintroducing gluten and dairy is slow and systematic. This is a unique chance to really see how your body tolerates these high-sensitivity foods. We want to add these foods to your diet responsibly and without compromising all your hard work. Here are the steps I recommend:

1. Start with dairy.
2. Eat it at least one serving two to three times a day for three days. Stick to plain milk or plain yogurt without anything added to see how you feel.
3. Track your response for the next seventy-two hours using the food log below.
4. If you have a reaction, stop dairy immediately.

DATE	FOOD REINTRODUCED	SYMPTOMS

Wait at least three days before testing gluten next. Follow these steps:

1. Eat foods containing gluten at least two to three times a day for three days. Use only plain wheat without added ingredients. The best thing to try is pasta, because most breads also contain yeast and sugar, or you might try cream of wheat cereal for breakfast.
2. Track your response for seventy-two hours using the food log below.
3. If you have a reaction, stop gluten immediately.

Tracking your symptoms and reactions is pretty straightforward. You can use the food log below to track your symptoms and monitor your progress. You can download it at www.10daydetox.com/resources and print out as many copies as you need to keep track of all your reactions as you transition off the program.

Every body is different, and everyone responds differently to food sensitivities. But to help you know what to be on the lookout for, here are some of the most common food-sensitivity reactions:

- Weight gain
- Resurgence of cravings
- Fluid retention
- Nasal congestion
- Headaches
- Brain fog
- Mood problems (depression, anxiety, anger, etc.)
- Sleep problems
- Joint aches
- Muscle aches
- Pain
- Fatigue
- Changes in your skin (acne, rashes, or eczema)
- Changes in digestion or bowel function (bloating, gas, diarrhea, constipation, reflux)

Gluten and dairy are by nature inflammatory (dairy may raise your insulin level even if you are not sensitive or allergic, so I recommend eating it only occasionally if you have diabesity). If you don't experience any reactions like the ones listed above within seventy-two hours, you should be safe and can freely incorporate the food.

In general, if you tolerate gluten and dairy, it is okay to eat them from time to time, but don't make them staples of your diet. For dairy choices, be sure to stay away from industrial processed cheese, as it is full of chemicals and additives and hormones. Also, modern forms of wheat (dwarf wheat) have much higher starch content and more gluten proteins, which make them more likely to cause inflammation. Try to find "heirloom" sources of gluten and dairy, such as grass-fed, heirloom cows and locally sourced cheeses. They may be more expensive, but they taste better and it will take less of them to satisfy your appetite.

You can also experiment with other grains such as spelt, rye, or Kamut. If you are not gluten sensitive, whole-kernel German rye bread can be a wonderful addition to your diet. Or try the "new" Einkorn wheat eaten by the ancient Sumerians. It is what we ate for thousands of years before hybridization led to the modern-day Frankenwheat we eat now. (This "new and improved" dwarf wheat has led to a 400 percent increase in celiac disease and caused 7 percent of the population to have gluten sensitivity.)

If you do experience a reaction, I recommend entirely eliminating the offending food from your diet for twelve weeks. For most people, this is enough time to allow the inflammation to cool. After that, you likely will once again be able to consume that food in small doses because the elapsed time will have allowed your leaky gut to heal. Still, I suggest limiting any problem food to once or twice a week so you don't trigger the same cycle of illness.

Often, it is one primary problem food, either gluten or dairy, that triggers the leaky gut, and then you react to a lot of other foods. If you stay off gluten and dairy, you can often include other foods you once reacted to without having problems. In other words, once you remove the primary triggers, the other allergens simply won't affect you as much. Again, though, I suggest limiting any potentially problematic foods to just once or twice a week so you don't trigger the same cycle of illness.

If you still react after eliminating that food for twelve weeks, avoid that food entirely, or see a physician, dietician, or nutritionist skilled in managing food allergies.

Reintroducing Treats

On the Blood Sugar Solution Plan for Life, you can add back in a few treats (such as coffee or tea, alcohol, and sweets) if you choose, but all in moderation and as an occasional pleasure, not a staple of everyday life. You can find some healthier sweets and treats in *The Blood Sugar Solution Cookbook*. Some people tolerate coffee or tea just fine, so I am least worried about that, but alcohol and sugar can be awful triggers for weight gain and out-of-control eating behaviors. Remember, they hijack your brain chemistry—so please be careful. Pay attention and track your responses. If you notice that cravings get triggered, it's a sign to scale back on the treats.

CHECKLIST FOR THE TRANSITION PHASE

- Do your personal "exit interview" in your Detox Journal.
- Choose the transition plan that best suits your needs.
- Continue with your daily practices of physical exercise, supplements, breathing exercises, UltraDetox Bath, journaling, tracking results, hydration, and seven to eight hours sleep.
- Fill out the "after" section of the Toxicity Questionnaire on pages 5–7.
- Redo your basic lab tests six weeks from the date you started the 10-Day Detox. Refer to the free guide *How to Work with Your Doctor to Get What You Need* for the right tests at www.10daydetox.com/resources.
- Continue to notice and track your diet, feelings, weight, waist size, hips, thighs, blood pressure, and blood sugar. You can track them once a week and keep aware of how you are feeling and what is changing. Plus, you'll easily be able to catch yourself if you're sliding.
- Stay connected to your buddy, your own small group, or the Blood Sugar Solution 10-Day Detox Diet online community by joining at www.10daydetox.com/resources.

PART VI

IT'S BIGGER THAN US

19

Getting Healthy Is a Team Sport

In Part I, I talked about the bigger issues that are contributing to our obesity and health crises. Our first order of business was to get *you* healthy and help you break free of food addiction. Now that we've gotten you on track, it will take a bigger effort from all of us combined to take back not just our own health, but also the health of our families and society. Think big here, because together, with our collective will and action, we can address the deeper challenges that created the health and weight problems in the first place. Together, we can fix our big fat global problem and make our world safer and healthier for ourselves and our children. Getting healthy is indeed a team sport!

Imagine if we lived in an environment where health wasn't something we had to "protect," but rather something that was the expected norm. Sadly, we have come to accept obesity as the new normal. I was recently looking at some family pictures and saw pictures of my grandmother Mary, who we also called fat Grandma Mary. Although she might have been technically overweight, by today's standards, she looks pretty normal. When I was a kid, I remember going to the carnival and seeing the "fat" lady, who weighed in at 300 pounds (136 kg). Now we see 300-pound people everywhere we go. Just go to McDonald's, or the supermarket, or the fairgrounds.

At Saddleback Church in California, where we created the healthy living program called the Daniel Plan, the average weight for women was 170 pounds (77 kg) and the average weight for men was 210 pounds (95 kg). And that was *average!*

This shift has happened over twenty or thirty years, almost without our noticing. It is said that if you place a frog in a pot of boiling water, it will jump right out. But if you put a frog in cold water and turn up the heat and slowly boil the water, the frog will cook to death. We are like those frogs, slowly coming to a boil in a similarly intolerable situation. We accept seat belt extenders as normal on airplanes. We accept super-size portions as standard options. Why is the smallest soda at a movie theater thirty-two ounces?

We have to begin challenging the idea that all this is normal and acceptable.

Diabesity is now our single biggest public health problem at home and abroad. Today, the leading cause of death in the developing world is not infectious disease or starvation, but obesity-related chronic disease. It kills 50 million people a year; that's twice the number of people who die from infection or starvation.

Why should we care about this? For so many reasons, not the least of which is that economic issues related to the obesity epidemic pose huge problems for us and for our children's future. One in five dollars of our gross national product goes to pay for health care costs caused mostly by diabesity, and the amount is growing by the day. These costs are the single biggest driver of our national debt. It's why we have had to mort-gage our future and why China owns much of our national debt.

The obesity epidemic threatens our global economic competitive-ness and national security. It undermines our ability to manage our federal debt, to educate and maintain a healthy and productive work force, and to maintain a viable military (up to 70 percent of military recruits are refused for service because they are too fat to fight).

On the home front, we have a choice about the kind of food envi-ronment we create today for children. Our children's future depends on turning the tide *now* for how food is made and sold in this country. We want to leave a legacy of health and well-being—not toxicity and chemically induced food addiction.

So what can you do to help fight back against the industrial food system? A lot! Here are some important strategies for becoming a game changer in the worldwide effort to take back our collective health.

GAME CHANGER #1: BE A VOICE FOR SOCIAL REFORM

Now that you know the truth—that food addiction is a social problem—you understand that we need social reform to set things right. Public health interventions are needed to protect the public, and we accept them all the time: seat belt laws, vaccination laws, smoking and alcohol regulations and taxes, food safety laws, elimination of leaded gas and paint. When the science has proven that processed food and especially sugar are addictive, it changes the conversation. When your brain is on drugs, willpower and personal responsibility are a fiction.

The sticking point is that the government doesn't want to get on the bad side of the one-trillion-dollar food industry. There's a reason that Michelle Obama agreed to call her campaign to fight childhood obesity "Let's Move." It was pressure from the food industry to not point fingers at food; they are stuck on the old mantra that there are no good or bad foods. The name "Let's Move" implies that the solution to our kids' problems lies simply in more exercise, and not in changing our food environment. And while the program itself does address changes in diet, including the need to improve the food in schools, those recommendations don't go nearly far enough. In fact, she partnered with the food industry to take 1.5 trillion calories out of the American diet. Sounds great, right? But this was accomplished by making Oreo cookies 90 instead of 100 calories, or cutting 15 calories out of a Pop Tart. It seems the message got coopted and the initiative got subverted. Oreos and Pop Tarts and all the other junk is still junk, even if it has a few less calories.

Everyone—including the Food and Drug Administration, the Department of Agriculture, and the surgeon general's office—is pussyfooting around and not calling out the food industry for loading us up with sugar. They all talk about "making better choices" and getting more exercise. But this approach unfairly blames the victims of a toxic food environment in which it is hard for most people to find real, fresh food.

We live in a toxic food landscape with tantalizing, addictive choices everywhere we go. The food industry justifies its production of toxic, addictive food by saying "We are just producing what our customers want." Of course they are. If they sold $2.99 bags of cocaine, a lot of customers would want that, too!

Fast-food and convenience stores far outnumber supermarkets and produce markets in most areas of the country. There is something called the Retail Food Environment Index (RFEI), which measures food deserts. It is the number of fast-food and convenience stores divided by the number of supermarkets and produce markets. In some parts of the country, that junk-to-real-food ratio is more than 10 to 1.

Michael Bloomberg, the former mayor of New York City, who didn't need or take money from interest groups to get elected, took a tough stand on changing the food environment so that it was more conducive to health. He implemented, among other things, smoking bans in public places and bans on trans fats. While his attempts to stop food stamp use for soda and to implement a soda tax were thwarted by the food industry, he brought national attention to this issue by trying to limit the sizes of soda sold in certain places. He might not have been able to accomplish all of his goals, but his efforts were enormously successful in raising public awareness about the insanity of our current food environment—and about who is really running the show.

Nobody wants government interference unless it is necessary to protect the health and welfare of its citizens. Nobody wants a nanny state telling us what to eat or how to live. But in fact, that is what we do have—just in reverse, with government policies that support, protect, and aid the one-trillion-dollar food industry rather than its people.

Detoxing our world requires widespread social and policy changes that make it easier to be healthy than to be sick or fat. There are many, many ways to start to reverse the national spiral of food addiction and obesity. Research has shown that public health education is necessary but not sufficient. Despite ongoing education and awareness of the dangers of sugar and industrial food, our health declines and our waistlines grow.

Changing the toxic food environment so people have better choices is a major requirement. If you go to the movies and the smallest soda is thirty-two ounces, how is that a choice? Especially when studies show that people will eat whatever is put in front of them, no matter the size. Given what we know now about the addictive nature of sugar and especially of sugar-sweetened and artificially sweetened beverages, we can no longer hide from or ignore this problem.

The more informed you are about what's going on and what can (and should) be done, the more voices we can lend to the global cause of fighting back. Learn as much as you can about what's going on behind the scenes in our food environment that directly affects your and your family's health and well-being. Write to your congressperson and senator and the White House. Write or e-mail the specific agencies in charge of food policy (the USDA, the FDA, and the Federal Trade Commission, or FTC). Use www.change.org to start a petition on any one of the topics below and make your voice heard.

Here are the changes that I believe we, as a country, should be striving for, to stop the babysitting of the food industry and start safeguarding the health of our families and citizens:

1. **Start a petition to change the name of the Farm Bill to the Food Bill,** because that's what it is. And stop subsidizing prices and profits for corn and soy that are turned into the high-fructose corn syrup and trans fats used to make sodas and processed food.

2. **Write to Congress demanding that every Farm Bill program that provides food to the poor and underserved (those**

most at risk for obesity) meet the highest nutritional standards and science of optimal nutrition. This goes for the food stamp or Supplemental Nutrition Assistance Program (SNAP), Women, Infants, and Children food program (WIC), Emergency Food Assistance Program, and the National School Lunch Program. The 2012 guidelines for the school lunch program required limits on saturated fat, sodium, calories, and trans fats, but there was no mention of sugar, even though the average teenager consumes about thirty teaspoons of sugar a day, or the equivalent of two 20-ounce sodas a day.

3. Call for the FDA to change the status of high-fructose corn syrup from GRAS (generally regarded as safe) to unsafe in currently consumed amounts. It is not safe in normally consumed amounts (about 15 percent of our total calories).

4. Advocate for the government to support the 2002 recommendations by the World Health Organization (WHO) and United Nations as detailed in a report called "Diet, Nutrition and the Prevention of Chronic Diseases," which calls for a limit on sugar to no more than 10 percent of total calories in the diet. In 2004, the WHO received a letter from the Bush administration stating that there was no evidence that fruits and vegetables prevented disease or that energy-dense, sugar-rich foods or fast foods contributed to obesity. No evidence?? The message from the government here was clear: "Don't confuse me with the facts, my mind's made up." The Bush administration, under pressure from the food lobby, threatened that if the report was published, the US would withhold its $406-million contribution to the WHO.

5. Demand that the food stamp, or SNAP, program no longer cover the purchase of sodas. Our government pays $4 billion a year to buy sodas for the poor with food stamps. That translates into 29 million servings of soda a day, or 10 billion servings a year to the poor, who suffer disproportionately from obesity, diabetes, and chronic disease and drive significant health care costs. Our government pays for soda on the front end and health care on the back end through Medicaid and Medicare.

6. **Lobby for the White House not to sign the "Cheeseburger Bill," also called the "American Personal Responsibility in Food Consumption Act,"** which would protect the food industry from lawsuits for harm caused by their products. Isn't the government's role to protect its citizens, not corporations?

7. **Insist that the government block the "Protecting Foods and Beverages from Government Attack Act of 2012,"** which would prohibit the use of federal money for public health campaigns against soda and other processed foods proven to cause obesity and disease.

8. **Support a Federal Trade Commission ban on all sugar and processed food marketing to children.** The FTC should revisit its 1972 prosecution of the sugar industry for promoting harmful, deceptive ads. The health ministers of fifty-two nations met and agreed to ban the marketing of junk food to children. Congress threatened to defund the FTC unless it stopped attempting to prevent junk food advertising to children. The US and Syria are among the few nations that allow this type of marketing to kids. Not great company. This is a no-brainer. We banned the marketing of alcohol and tobacco to kids, and it made a difference. Yet your kids still see 30,000 commercials a year for junk food. As a parent, you can't compete with that kind of propaganda.

9. **Write to the FDA requesting that food labels be fixed to reflect the true quality of the food.** The "traffic light" method of green, yellow, and red that is used in other countries makes it simple to understand labels and choose food based on the science of how it affects your health. Green is healthy and can be eaten freely. Yellow should be eaten with caution and moderately. And red means eat at your own risk! Food label guidelines, created by the Food and Drug Administration, are heavily influenced by food industry lobbyists and are designed

to confuse consumers by making it unclear whether something is good or bad for you unless you have a PhD in nutrition science.

10. **Write to Congress to end the conflict of interest. Remove responsibility for food policy and dietary recommendations from the USDA.** They support agriculture, not health. It's like putting the fox in charge of the hen house. These responsibilities should be turned over to the Department of Health and Human Services or a newly formed food agency that does not have the USDA's inherent conflict of interest.

11. **Lobby Congress to tax soda and sugar-sweetened beverages.** They are the largest source of sugar calories in our diet and the ones most strongly linked by science to obesity and diabetes. The revenues from this tax could be funneled back into proven obesity-fighting programs for the poor and underserved. This strategy worked with alcohol and tobacco. And if the soda lobby thought this move would *not* have a significant impact on soda consumption, it would not spend over $20 million a year to fight it, or give $10 million to the City of Philadelphia to stop the law by supporting an obesity program at the Children's Hospital.

12. **Contact your local zoning regulators and work together to support restrictions on access to sugar.** This can be done by limiting the number and density of convenience stores and fast-food outlets (improving the Retail Food Environment Index), especially in low-income neighborhoods and around schools, and providing incentives for grocery stores and farmers' markets. There are programs now that double the value of food stamp dollars used at farmers' markets. We could also institute age limits (such as a minimum age of eighteen) for the purchase of drinks with added sugar, just as we do for alcohol.

These are just starter ideas. I have written more about how we can all "Take Back Our Health" in *The Blood Sugar Solution*. And in the next few suggestions, you will learn more about what you can do at home and in your community to personally influence social reform. You can also share your ideas at www.takebackourhealth.org.

GAME CHANGER #2: REDESIGN YOUR WORLD FOR HEALTH

While it hasn't been proven that more parks and sidewalks lead to a skinnier population, we do know that your immediate environment plays a big role in your health. Remember Dan Buettner's experiment in Minnesota, where he implemented changes in the environment that led to significant weight loss and health? Kids lost 10 percent of their body weight after eating in classrooms and hallways was prohibited. And the town lost 12,000 pounds (5,500 kg) by having residents agree to use ten-inch plates and having grocers put healthy foods at the checkout counters. Your environment *does* matter.

Imagine if your health bubble extended way beyond the boundaries of your own personal environment. Imagine if you could help build and create a world where healthy choices were not just available, but easy and *automatic*.

Here are just a few ways you can begin to change the infrastructure for health:

1. **Take back school lunchrooms.** The Healthy, Hunger-Free Kids Act of 2010, which removes junk food from schools and supports access to fresh produce through farm-to-school networks, is a great start, but we need more—much more. For ideas on what you can do to get involved, I recommend watching the documentary *Two Angry Moms* or reading the companion book, *Lunch Wars*.

2. **Band together with other parents and rally your school administrators** to support "eat only in lunchroom" policies and the integration of nutrition and cooking skills into the curriculum (then think bigger and lobby your local politicians to support changes in

zoning laws to prevent fast-food and junk-food retailers from operating near schools!). Andrea Ryan, the wife of Tim Ryan, the congressman from Ohio who wrote *A Mindful Nation*, is a fourth-grade teacher. She allows her kids to eat food in class only if it is a raw fruit or vegetable — so the kids demand that their parents buy them more fruits and vegetables. One teacher, one class, but this is something that is scalable to every school.

3. **Visit your local grocer and ask for healthier items.** Merchandisers will respond to the requests of their consumers, and if enough people start asking, they will catch on. One crusader I know goes around the grocery store moving the healthy stuff to shelves at eye level to give it better visual placement.

4. **Suggest healthy options to your favorite local restaurants.** The more these items are requested, the more likely they are to show up on the menu as everyday choices.

5. **Talk to your human resources department** about improving the food culture at your workplace by offering healthier alternatives in the lunchroom or vending machines, and during meetings or other company events.

6. **Work with administrators at your place of worship** to ensure that there are healthy foods and beverages at gatherings and events. You can also create fitness activities to do together at your place of worship; take a look at www.danielplan.com for more ideas and examples. You can also start the Daniel Plan at your place of worship. We have created a whole curriculum to make it easy to get started.

GAME CHANGER #3: TELL A FRIEND

After you experience a health transformation yourself, you will likely want to share your newly discovered insights and passion, which is great. But tread lightly — no one wants to be lectured to! Instead, you can share by example. Getting healthy yourself will cause people to wonder how you did it. In the course of your everyday life, as you change your small daily habits (for instance, ordering herbal tea instead of a latte when meeting friends for coffee, or bringing nuts or fresh veggies and homemade dip for a workday snack instead of raiding the vending machine), people will naturally be curious. When they ask about your new lifestyle, take the opportunity to pass along the food-addiction and detox secrets you now know. If you do this with respect (and not judgment), others will likely want to know more and be receptive to learning the real facts. Even if you open the eyes of *one* person, you've paid it forward and made a difference.

Better yet, encourage your friends to join you. Invite them to go shopping with you, to cook and enjoy a meal together. Start a group at work or in your community for people who want to take back their health and go on hikes, play games or sports together, and have dinners. Start a supper club. Start a church group. Start a friendly competition at work and see who can get the healthiest by dejunking their work spaces, or form teams and see who can lose the most weight, walk the most steps, or eat the most vegetables in a week. Remember the words of Margaret Mead: *"Never doubt that a small group of thoughtful, committed citizens can change the world. Indeed, it is the only thing that ever has."*

GAME CHANGER #4: VOTE WITH YOUR WALLET

The single most powerful weapon you have to take down the food industry is your wallet. Your dollars are what the food industry is after; how you spend them dictates *everything!* Think about it: Where does the $1 trillion we spend on factory-made hyperprocessed junk and fast food come from? It comes from us—from our wallets and paychecks. While asking for policy, industrial, and social reform is important, the truth is *we*—not the government or corporations—already hold the keys to fixing this.

Imagine if we just stopped buying the food industry's unhealthy products, even for a day. If we refused to buy these processed and addictive foods, the industry would lose its major source of profits, and we would collectively make a difference in what appears on our grocery shelves.

We could change how our food is grown and produced, stop the destruction of our soils and depletion of our natural aquifers, and transform agriculture from an oil-based industry (one that uses more fossil fuels than all our cars put together) into a more sustainable, local, health-creating, and community-building food system. We could renew our oceans and estuaries destroyed by the runoff from factory farms. We could end climate change by closing factory animal farms, which create clouds of methane gas (a bigger contributor to global warming than carbon dioxide).

What you choose to purchase and put on your fork is the ultimate game changer. It is the most important thing you can do for yourself, your family, your community, our nation, and the planet. Period!

GAME CHANGER #5: EAT AT HOME

Where you eat may be just as important as *what* you eat. Not only does this make an impact in terms of where our dollars are spent—it puts the control over what goes in your food squarely in your hands. A hundred years ago, only 2 percent of our meals were eaten outside the home. Today, that number has escalated to 50 percent. I believe in the power of collective intelligence, and as more and more families wake up to the power of taking back their kitchens, we'll turn the tide.

Imagine an experiment. Or better yet, let's call it a celebration: We'll call upon the people of the world to join together and celebrate eating whole, real, fresh food at home for one week. I call it an eat-in, like the nonviolent sit-in protests of the 1960s, but the eat-in won't get you arrested! For one week (or even one day!), we all eat breakfast and dinner at home with our families or friends. Imagine the power of all those forks to change the world.

The extraordinary thing is that we really do have the ability to influence large corporations and social change by our collective choices. We can reclaim the family dinner. Doing so will reinforce how easy it is to find and prepare real food quickly and simply, and teach our children by example how to connect, build security, and develop social skills—meal after meal, day after day, year after year.

I recently went to South Carolina to help an obese family as part of a film on childhood obesity called *Fed Up*. The family was massively overweight. The father was in dialysis but couldn't get a kidney transplant because of his weight, and the son at sixteen was 260 pounds (118 kg) and 60 percent body fat.

They lived on food stamps and disability. Instead of a prescription, I brought them the Environmental Working Group's (EWG) guide *Good Food on a Tight Budget* and groceries for turkey chili, roasted sweet potatoes, and a salad and went to their trailer and taught them to cook a meal.

I left them with the EWG's guide to eating well for less and my *Blood Sugar Solution Cookbook* and suggested they cook and eat at home using the guide. After five months, the mother lost 57 pounds (26 kg) and the father and son each lost 40 pounds (18 kg). Now the father can get a new kidney. It is a myth that eating well and cooking real food from real ingredients is too hard, takes too much time, and is too expensive. Nonsense. If a family of five on food stamps can do it, anyone can.

We can take back our kitchens one family at a time, one home at a time. We can take back our health.

Here are some tips that will help you take back the family dinner in your home, starting today:

1. **Prioritize cooking.** It is the essential act that makes us human and is vital for our own health and our family's and community's health, but it also connects us to nature and the larger community. We have to cook our way out of this mess of obesity and disease. Spending time preparing our own food is a simple but transformational act.

2. **Keep your pantry and fridge clean.** Keep out any food with high-fructose corn syrup or hydrogenated fats, or with sugar listed as

the first or second ingredient on the label. Fill your cabinets and fridge with real, fresh, whole foods. For a full refresher on the kitchen makeover, see page 98 in "The Prep Phase."

3. **Read Laurie David's book** *The Family Dinner.* She suggests simple but effective guidelines, such as scheduling a set dinnertime, banning phones and other devices from the dinner table, turning off the television, serving everyone the same meal, cleaning up together, and more.

4. **Eat together.** No matter how modest the meal, savor the ritual of the table. Sit down together and treat one another and your food with care and respect. Mealtime is a time to communicate and nourish ourselves on every level. Say a blessing of gratitude before your meal. Use a traditional blessing or make one up that is unique to your family and friends!

GAME CHANGER #6: GET INVOLVED IN YOUR COMMUNITY

People helping people works. Community-based models, like the one we created for the Daniel Plan, have shown up in other forms across the globe. Peers for Progress created pilot programs based on peer support to treat diabetes in Cameroon, Uganda, Thailand, and South Africa. The peer support group models were more effective than conventional-care interventions for improving the health of diabetics, and health care costs decreased tenfold. In Thailand, a community garden is irrigated by an old bike hooked up to a generator run by patients with diabetes. They get exercise and grow their own healthy food at the same time!

An old African proverb says that if you want to travel swiftly, travel alone, but if you want to travel far, travel together. There are many, many ways you can help bring together people on the path to health beyond even the small, personal groups you've established as part of the Blood Sugar Solution 10-Day Detox community.

Here are just a few ideas to get you started:

1. **Put out a call for healthy recipes to your friends and family** and collect them in a community cookbook. One mom did this within her child's grade school; she collected over fifty healthy recipes and created a PDF that the entire parent body and teachers now share.

2. **Plant a community garden.** This is a great way to bring people together and grow the most delicious, nutritious, and environmentally friendly food imaginable.

3. **Talk to your human resources department at work** about training wellness champions in the workplace. These people (meaning you!) can lead support groups for others to get healthy by following the Blood Sugar Solution 10-Day Detox Diet or doing the online course together (see www.10daydetox.com/resources).

4. **Establish a CSA (community-supported agriculture group) or farmers' market** in your town. Check out www.localharvest.org or go to www.10daydetox.com/resources for information on how.

5. **Start a hiking or walking group,** or organize a weekly bike ride. Combining friends and fitness is a great way to make exercise easy and fun.

6. **Start a men's group or a women's group**—or really, just start any group to get people together to focus on healthy living and fulfillment. It could be breakfast once a week at a diner willing to accommodate your healthy preferences, or coffee (hopefully decaf!) one afternoon, or anything that gives continuity, support, and meaning through connection.

7. **Volunteer.** The simple act of giving to others satisfies a human need to be of service, and also provides deep happiness. Getting out of our own world and into someone else's connects us to our common humanity. Science shows that altruism activates the same reward pathways in the brain as sugar, but without all the bad side effects.

8. **Get involved with your local schools.** If you have kids, work with the schools to improve the food (see the movie *Lunch Wars* or visit www.angrymoms.org). If you don't have kids, help them plant a garden, teach meditation, or run a healthy bake sale. Find a way to share your unique gifts and skills.

Obesity, diabetes, and food addiction are social diseases, and we need a social cure. My personal hope is that together we can create a national conversation and a movement about real, practical solutions for the prevention, treatment, and reversal of our big fat problem. But you can start with you, your family, and your community. The health of our world and our future depends on it.

PART VII

THE 10-DAY DETOX MEAL PLAN AND RECIPES

20

The Meal Plan

Let's get cooking!

But first, just a quick recap of your options for the 10-Day Detox. There are two recipe plans to choose from: the *Core Plan* and the *Adventure Plan*. Meals on the Core Plan are very simple yet healthy, and can be made by everyone—even cooking novices. Remember, if you can read, you can cook!

For those of you who have more time and want to experiment with some new flavors, the Adventure Plan takes the fun one step further.

You should feel free to mix and match between the two plans, as long as you pick all of your meals for any given day from that day's Core and Adventure plans; don't pick lunches and dinners from different days. The daily menus are carefully balanced to make sure you get the right dose of nutrients.

Lastly, you always have the option to prepare a basic protein and nonstarchy vegetable for lunch or dinner. I've given you everything you need to know to make these super-simple meals in the "Cooking the Basics" section on pages 258–61.

On page 257, you will find the 10-Day Detox Staples Shopping List, which includes the kitchen essentials that will enable you to make a variety of healthy meals, both during these ten days and after. I also encourage you to read through the 10-Day Meal Plan in advance and choose your meals, so you can shop ahead for the specific ingredients you will need for those recipes.

"WILL I BE HUNGRY?"

The answer to that is short and simple: NO! Remember, this program isn't about deprivation. The meals are all designed to ensure that your blood sugar is balanced and your stomach, and taste buds, are more than satisfied.

Having said that, I realize that each of you will have different caloric requirements. A six-foot-tall person who starts the program at 300 pounds (136 kg) will need more food than someone five feet four inches and 150 pounds (68 kg). The secret to making this meal plan work for you? Personalize it!

Use each recipe as a guide, but feel free to modify it with the whole foods listed in the guidelines below to meet your individual needs. Some of you will do just fine with the recipes as is, and some of you will need more food to achieve your daily goals of work, exercise, or normal metabolic function. I suggest starting the 10-Day Detox by following the recipes as written, and then after the first day or two, make any necessary adjustments. You'll know you need to eat more if you:

- Crave sweets between meals
- Get light-headed or fatigued between meals
- Can't make it through your thirty-minute walks
- Crave coffee to keep going or get started in the morning
- Have difficulty concentrating
- Feel moody, anxious, or short-tempered
- Experience common signs of hunger between meals, such as belly growling or a vacant sensation in the abdominal and chest area

If you feel you need to eat more, follow these guidelines:

- The recipes for the Breakfast Detox Shakes are designed for the average person. Only one problem: There is no such thing as an average person. I need a double portion because I have a good metabolism and am a very lean six feet three inches and 180 pounds (82 kg). If you feel

Nonstarchy Vegetables . . . Eat as Much as You Like!

Artichoke	Hearts of palm
Aubergine	Jalapeño peppers
Asparagus	Kale
Bean sprouts	Lettuces
Beet greens	Mushrooms
Bell peppers (red, yellow, green)	Mustard greens
Broccoli	Onions
Brussels sprouts	Parsley
Cabbage	Radicchio
Cauliflower	Radishes
Celery	Rocket
Chives	Shallots
Collard greens	Snow peas
Courgettes	Spinach
Dandelion greens	Sugar-snap peas
Endive	Summer squash
Fennel	Swiss chard
Garlic	Tomatoes
Ginger	Turnip greens
Green beans	Watercress

hungry, you can add extra nuts, coconut butter, or avocado to your shakes, or add a scoop of high-quality chia, hemp, or plant-based protein powder (unsweetened). You can also drink a bigger portion size. See how much you need to keep you satisfied until lunchtime.

- Add an extra 1 to 2 ounces of protein per meal at lunch and/or dinner. Remember to choose high-quality sources, such as poultry, omega-3 eggs, fish, tofu, or tempeh. If possible, choose wild, grass-fed, or organic versions (and non-GMO for tofu and tempeh).

- Eat as many nonstarchy vegetables as you want (see box on the previous page for the full list of options). Go crazy! Vegetables will keep you satiated longer and boost your detox process.
- Don't forget snacks! It's easy to forget these smaller meals if you are not used to snacking. I encourage you to take time to plan ahead for your two snacks per day. Eating a small protein-based snack with healthy fats and fiber, like nuts or the spreads listed in the recipes, will help keep your blood sugar steady and your energy up.

Your goal is to eat until you are gently satisfied. Trust your body and its instincts, and pay attention to what it is telling you. You'll know you ate more than your body needs if you feel stuffed. When in doubt, follow the Okinawan teaching of *hara hachi bu,* which advises us to eat until we are 80 percent full. Considering that Okinawans follow this closely and are among the longest-living people on the planet, that seems like sage advice.

YOUR DAILY MEALS

Each day, your meal plan consists of the following:

Breakfast

You can choose from any of the Breakfast Detox Shakes in the recipe section. I encourage you to try them all to find the ones you like best.

Lunch

In the Core Plan, you have two easy-to-prepare, super-healthy options you can make for lunch: soup, or Dr. Hyman's Super Salad Bar.

My Super Salad Bar enables you to assemble lunch in minutes by having fresh, delicious salad ingredients already prepped in your refrigerator.

If you have access to a kitchen to reheat soups during the day, you can choose any of the five delicious soup recipes. These broth-based soups are comforting and filling, and are great for those of you who like to be creative with your vegetable intake. They provide loads of fat-busting nutrients and energy to restore your vitality. Be sure to make enough so you can enjoy soup several times throughout the week; stored in sealed glass containers, these soups can last three to four days in the refrigerator (or up to six months in the freezer).

Both the salad and soup options need a satisfying serving of protein to go along with them to maintain your energy and maximize detoxification. **Be sure to add 4 to 6 ounces of protein of your choice** (when possible, use sustainably raised, grass-fed, or organic): chicken, turkey, salmon, omega-3 eggs, tofu, or tempeh, either mixed in or on the side (for simple protein preparation instructions, take a look at the "Cooking the Basics" section on pages 258–61). You can mix your salad ingredients in advance, put the protein and the dressing in separate containers, and bring it all to work. Toss together right before you are ready to eat; otherwise, your salad will be soggy.

Dinner

As with lunch, each day you can choose from the Core Plan or Adventure Plan dinner. Or, if you prefer, you can make a simple protein and vegetable according to the instructions in the "Cooking the Basics" section.

Whichever dinner option you choose, remember you can always augment with as many nonstarchy vegetables as you like. The more vegetables, the better.

10-DAY DETOX STAPLES SHOPPING LIST

The following is a list of the basics you should have in your kitchen to enable you to make a wide variety of healthy meals for these ten days—and long after. Some of these ingredients may not necessarily appear in the detox recipes, but they are great to have on hand for quick meals you can make according to the "Cooking the Basics" guidelines on page 258.

- Extra virgin olive oil
- Extra virgin coconut butter (often called coconut oil; at room temperature it is solid, but at warm temperatures it may be liquid)
- Other healthy oils that you like (walnut, sesame, grape seed, flax, or avocado)
- Nut butters (raw if possible; choose from almond, cashew, macadamia, or walnut)
- Nuts: walnuts, almonds, pecans, macadamia
- Seeds: hemp, chia, flax, pumpkin, sesame
- Tahini (sesame seed paste — great for salad dressings and in sauces for vegetables)
- Canned full fat coconut milk
- Unsweetened hemp or almond milk
- Canned or jarred Kalamata olives
- Ground almond
- Apple cider vinegar
- Balsamic vinegar
- Low-sodium, gluten-free tamari
- Low-sodium broth (vegetable or chicken)
- Dijon mustard
- Sea salt
- Black pepper (peppercorns that you can freshly grind)
- Detoxifying and anti-inflammatory herbs and spices, including turmeric, cayenne pepper, thyme, rosemary, chili powder, cumin, sage, oregano, onion powder, cinnamon, coriander, cilantro, paprika, and parsley

COOKING THE BASICS

Below are a few basic cooking techniques that will allow you to make quick meals if you choose to replace any of the lunches or dinners from the 10-Day Detox.

Cooking Vegetables

Steam or sauté your vegetables and add some fresh or dried herbs or spices.

To steam:

- In a large saucepan, bring 1 cup of water to a boil.
- Place a steaming rack or basket over the water (you can get one at any grocery store for about $2).
- Chop your veggies. Place them in the steaming rack, cover, and steam for 4 to 8 minutes, depending on the vegetable and your desired level of tenderness. They should still be crunchy and bright colored.
- Add your favorite seasonings and drizzle with olive oil and a little salt to taste. You can cook almost any vegetable this way. It's easy. It's delicious. And it takes almost no time at all.

To sauté:

- Chop your veggies.
- In a sauté pan, heat 1 tablespoon of extra virgin olive oil over medium-high heat.
- Add the veggies and sauté for 5 to 7 minutes, stirring occasionally, until they are cooked to your desired level of tenderness.
- You can add onions, garlic, and/or mushrooms (shiitake are particularly tasty) to sautéed veggies to make them more flavorful. You might want to sauté these vegetables with a little salt first, then add the others.

Cooking Fish and Chicken

Fish and chicken are easy to prepare in delicious and healthy ways. Just grill, broil, or sauté your fish or boneless, skinless chicken, then season with extra virgin olive oil, lemon juice, rosemary, garlic, ginger, or cilantro (I like to experiment with spices). Here's how:

To grill or broil:

- Prepare the grill or preheat the broiler.
- Sprinkle salt and any other seasoning you choose on your fish or chicken. You can coat it in 1 teaspoon of olive oil. Then place it on the grill or under the broiler.
- Cook fish until it is tender and opaque throughout, 7 to 10 minutes, flipping it once halfway through the cooking time. Chicken will take longer, perhaps up to 15 minutes. Again, flip it halfway. You'll know it's done if it's firm to the touch and white throughout when you slice it. You can use a meat thermometer to be sure, but after a while it will be second nature.

To sauté:

- Sprinkle salt and any other seasoning you choose on your fish or chicken.
- In a skillet or sauté pan, heat 1 to 2 tablespoons of extra virgin olive oil over medium-high heat. Add the fish or chicken to the pan.
- Turn fish just once while cooking, but turn chicken often to avoid browning it too much on one side. Follow the same cooking times as for broiling and grilling.
- You can sauté onions, garlic, mushrooms, or other vegetables with your fish or chicken to make it especially tasty.
- Once it is cooked, season fish or chicken with additional salt, freshly ground black pepper, up to 1 tablespoon of olive oil, and lemon juice if you choose.

Tofu or Tempeh

Follow the guidelines for fish and chicken, or simply add cubed tofu or tempeh to your vegetables before steaming or sautéing.

Spice Up Your Food

Remember to add herbs and spices to your cooking. Add fresh rosemary, chopped fresh cilantro, or fresh crushed garlic or fresh sliced ginger to your vegetables. Using either dried or fresh herbs adds flavor and incredible detoxification benefits. Place slices of ginger in the water while you're cooking rice (once you have transitioned off the 10-Day Detox), or add 1 to 2 teaspoons of turmeric for delicious yellow, Indian-style rice. These are powerful anti-inflammatories, and they give the rice a wonderful aroma and flavor. Try different cooking styles to add natural flavor as well. For example, roasting hearty vegetables such as Brussels sprouts or onions brings out their natural sweetness. There is a plethora of ways to eat your veggies—just keep trying new flavors, new prep styles, and different vegetables until you find what you like best. And remember, you can't overeat these foods, so eat all the broccoli and lettuce you want!

THE 10-DAY DETOX MEAL PLAN

Here is a recap of your 10-Day Detox Meal Plan:

Day 1

- Breakfast: Detox Shake of your choice (page 267)
- Midmorning Snack: 10 to 12 nuts (almonds, walnuts, pecans, macadamia nuts)
- Lunch:
  - Core Plan: Choice of soup with protein (page 273) or Dr. Hyman's Super Salad Bar with protein (page 271)
  - Adventure Plan: Kale and Red Cabbage Slaw with Turkey Meatballs (page 288)
- Midafternoon Snack: Dip or spread of your choice (page 316) with fresh vegetables
- Dinner:
  - Core Plan: Grilled Salmon with Onion Marmalade over Greens (page 277)
  - Adventure Plan: Coconut Curry with Fish or Tofu (page 300)

Day 2

- Breakfast: Detox Shake (page 267)
- Midmorning Snack: 10 to 12 nuts (almonds, walnuts, pecans, macadamia nuts)
- Lunch:
  - Core Plan: Soup with protein (page 273) or Dr. Hyman's Super Salad Bar with protein (page 271)
  - Adventure Plan: Bok Choy Salad with Tofu or Raw Almonds (page 289)
- Midafternoon Snack: Dip or spread of your choice (page 316) with fresh vegetables
- Dinner:
  - Core Plan: Grilled Snapper with Salad (page 278)
  - Adventure Plan: Chicken Breast with Ratatouille and Steamed Broccoli (page 302)

Day 3

- Breakfast: Detox Shake (page 267)
- Midmorning Snack: 10 to 12 nuts (almonds, walnuts, pecans, macadamia nuts)
- Lunch:
  - Core Plan: Soup with protein (page 273) or Dr. Hyman's Super Salad Bar with protein (page 271)
  - Adventure Plan: Walnut Pâté with Fresh Tomato Salsa (page 290)
- Midafternoon Snack: Dip or spread of your choice (page 316) with fresh vegetables
- Dinner:
  - Core Plan: Asian-Flavored Chicken Skewers with Wilted Leafy Greens (pages 279–80)
  - Adventure Plan: Grilled Salmon or Tofu Vegetable Kebabs (page 304)

Day 4

- Breakfast: Detox Shake (page 267)
- Midmorning Snack: 10 to 12 nuts (almonds, walnuts, pecans, macadamia nuts)
- Lunch:
  - Core Plan: Soup with protein (page 273) or Dr. Hyman's Super Salad Bar with protein (page 271)
  - Adventure Plan: Cod Cakes over Mixed Greens (page 295)
- Midafternoon Snack: Dip or spread of your choice (page 316) with fresh vegetables
- Dinner:
  - Core Plan: Stir-Fry Vegetables with Almonds (page 284)
  - Adventure Plan: Bibimbap-Style Vegetables with Egg or Tofu in Spicy Chili Sauce (page 310)

Day 5

- Breakfast: Detox Shake (page 267)
- Midmorning Snack: 10 to 12 nuts (almonds, walnuts, pecans, macadamia nuts)
- Lunch:
  - Core Plan: Soup with protein (page 273) or Dr. Hyman's Super Salad Bar with protein (page 271)
  - Adventure Plan: Vegetable Rolls with Shredded Chicken and Nut Cream (page 291)
- Midafternoon Snack: Dip or spread of your choice (page 316) with fresh vegetables
- Dinner:
  - Core Plan: Herb-Crusted Chicken Breasts with Roasted Garlic (page 281)
  - Adventure Plan: Roast Fish Casserole with Fennel and Leeks (page 306)

Day 6

- Breakfast: Detox Shake (page 267)
- Midmorning Snack: 10 to 12 nuts (almonds, walnuts, pecans, macadamia nuts)
- Lunch:
  - Core Plan: Soup with protein (page 273) or Dr. Hyman's Super Salad Bar with protein (page 271)
  - Adventure Plan: Chopped Vegetable Salad with Salmon (page 293)
- Midafternoon Snack: Dip or spread of your choice (page 316) with fresh vegetables
- Dinner:
  - Core Plan: Baked Cod with Olive and Caper Pesto (page 282)
  - Adventure Plan: Almond–Flax Crusted Chicken (page 307)

Day 7

- Breakfast: Detox Shake (page 267)
- Midmorning Snack: 10 to 12 nuts (almonds, walnuts, pecans, macadamia nuts)
- Lunch:
  - Core Plan: Soup with protein (page 273) or Dr. Hyman's Super Salad Bar with protein (page 271)
  - Adventure Plan: Cucumber Salad with Sunflower Mock Tuna (page 294)
- Midafternoon Snack: Dip or spread of your choice (page 316) with fresh vegetables
- Dinner:
  - Core Plan: Roast Chicken Breast with Rosemary (page 283)
  - Adventure Plan: Beef with Bok Choy (page 308)

Day 8

- Breakfast: Detox Shake (page 267)

- Midmorning Snack: 10 to 12 nuts (almonds, walnuts, pecans, macadamia nuts)
- Lunch:
  - Core Plan: Soup with protein (page 273) or Dr. Hyman's Super Salad Bar with protein (page 271)
  - Adventure Plan: Arugula, Avocado, and Grilled Snapper (page 296)
- Midafternoon Snack: Dip or spread of your choice (page 316) with fresh vegetables
- Dinner:
  - Core Plan: Grilled Pepper Steak (page 285)
  - Adventure Plan: Chicken Breast Stuffed with Sun-Dried Tomato Pesto, with Sautéed Spinach (page 312)

Day 9

- Breakfast: Detox Shake (page 267)
- Midmorning Snack: 10 to 12 nuts (almonds, walnuts, pecans, macadamia nuts)
- Lunch:
  - Core Plan: Soup with protein (page 273) or Dr. Hyman's Super Salad Bar with protein (page 271)
  - Adventure Plan: Spiced Turkey Wrap with Watercress and Avocado (page 298)
- Midafternoon Snack: Dip or spread of your choice (page 316) with fresh vegetables
- Dinner:
  - Core Plan: Steamed Snapper with Ginger and Scallions (page 286)
  - Adventure Plan: Thai Fish Salad (page 313)

Day 10

- Breakfast: Detox Shake (page 267)
- Midmorning Snack: 10 to 12 nuts (almonds, walnuts, pecans, macadamia nuts)

- Lunch:
  - Core Plan: Soup with protein (page 273) or Dr. Hyman's Super Salad Bar with protein (page 271)
  - Adventure Plan: Watercress and Arugula Salad with Poached Eggs (page 299)
- Midafternoon Snack: Dip or spread of your choice (page 316) with fresh vegetables
- Dinner:
  - Core Plan: Grilled Tofu with Cilantro Pesto (page 286)
  - Adventure Plan: Chicken Encrusted with Red Chili Pesto (page 315)

21

The Recipes

Food should be delightful, delicious, and nourishing to body, mind, and soul. These recipes are all designed to create pleasure and vibrant health. Enjoy!

BREAKFAST DETOX SHAKES

DR. HYMAN'S WHOLE-FOOD PROTEIN SHAKE

Serves: 1 Prep time: 5 minutes

- 75 g frozen blueberries
- 50 g frozen cranberries
- ¼ organic lemon with the rind (optional)
- 1 tablespoon almond butter
- 1 tablespoon pumpkin seeds (see note overleaf)
- 1 tablespoon chia seeds (see note overleaf)
- 1 tablespoon hemp seeds (see note overleaf)
- 2 raw walnuts (see note overleaf)
- 2 raw Brazil nuts (see note overleaf)
- ¼ avocado
- ½ tablespoon extra virgin coconut butter
- 120 ml unsweetened almond or hemp milk
- 120 ml water

Combine all the ingredients in a blender and blend on high speed until smooth. You can also whiz all the ingredients in a wide-necked Mason jar using a hand-held blender and drink the shake right from the jar. Be sure to add enough water so that the smoothie is drinkable but still thick (total liquid should be 2 to 3 cm above the other ingredients before blending). You can also make it thicker and eat it with a spoon.

NOTE: To activate the enzymes in the seeds and nuts in any smoothie recipe for easier digestion, you can soak them ahead of time. Fill a bowl with enough water to cover the seeds or nuts and soak for at least 30 minutes, preferably overnight if time permits.

Nutritional analysis per serving (375 ml): calories 547, fat 52 g, saturated fat 10 g, cholesterol 0 mg, fiber 13 g, protein 15 g, carbohydrate 27 g, sodium 41 mg

KIWI AND CHIA SEED SMOOTHIE

Serves: 1 Prep time: 5 minutes
- 1 kiwi fruit (slightly firm), peeled and cut in half
- ¼ avocado
- 4 tablespoons chia seeds (see note below)
- juice of ½ lime
- 5 g fresh mint leaves
- 4 to 5 ice cubes (optional)
- 220 ml water
- 30 g spinach or 1 medium kale leaf, stem removed

Combine all the ingredients in a blender and blend on high speed until smooth.

NOTE: To activate the enzymes in the seeds and nuts in any smoothie recipe for easier digestion, you can soak them ahead of time. Fill a bowl with enough water to cover the seeds or nuts and soak for at least 30 minutes, preferably overnight if time permits.

Nutritional analysis per serving (400 ml): calories 265, fat 18 g, saturated fat 2 g, cholesterol 0 mg, fiber 18 g, protein 10 g, carbohydrate 31 g, sodium 58 mg

GINGER AND CUCUMBER SMOOTHIE

Serves: 1 Prep time: 5 minutes

- 75 g raw almonds (see note below)
- 2 kale leaves, stems removed
- 4 tablespoons chia seeds (see note below)
- 1 cm piece fresh root ginger, peeled
- ½ medium cucumber, peeled and seeded
- 250 ml water (or more for desired thickness)

Combine all the ingredients in a blender and blend on high speed until smooth.

NOTE: To activate the enzymes in the seeds and nuts in any smoothie recipe for easier digestion, you can soak them ahead of time. Fill a bowl with enough water to cover the seeds or nuts and soak for at least 30 minutes, preferably overnight if time permits.

Nutritional analysis per serving (500 ml): calories 446, fat 34 g, saturated fat 3 g, cholesterol 0 mg, fiber 18 g, protein 19 g, carbohydrate 35 g, sodium 42 mg

SPICED ALMOND SMOOTHIE

Serves: 1 Prep time: 5 minutes

- 1 tablespoon raw almond butter
- ¼ avocado
- 1 kale leaf, stem removed
- ¼ cucumber, peeled
- ¼ lime, peeled and seeded
- 8 to 10 fresh mint leaves, chopped
- 1 cm piece fresh root ginger, peeled
- ½ teaspoon extra virgin coconut butter
- 40 g hemp seeds (see note below)
- 1 tablespoon chia seeds (see note below)
- 250 ml water
- 2 to 3 ice cubes, depending on how cold you like your drinks
- optional: ¼ jalapeño chili, seeds removed

Combine all the ingredients in a blender and blend on high speed until smooth.

NOTE: To activate the enzymes in the seeds and nuts in any smoothie recipe for easier digestion, you can soak them ahead of time. Fill a bowl with enough water to cover the seeds or nuts and soak for at least 30 minutes, preferably overnight if time permits.

Nutritional analysis per serving (500 ml): 437 calories, fat 35 g, saturated fat 5 g, cholesterol 0 mg, fiber 10 g, protein 18 g, carbohydrate 20 g, sodium 21 mg

ALMOND AND STRAWBERRY SMOOTHIE

Serves: 1 Prep time: 5 minutes
- 1 tablespoon raw almond butter
- 3 raw walnuts (see note below)
- 250 ml water
- 75 g fresh or frozen strawberries
- ¼ avocado
- 1 cm piece fresh root ginger, peeled
- ¼ teaspoon ground cinnamon
- 1 tablespoon flaxseeds (see note below)
- 2 to 3 ice cubes, depending on how cold you like your drinks

Combine all the ingredients in a blender and blend on high speed until smooth.

NOTE: To activate the enzymes in the seeds and nuts in any smoothie recipe for easier digestion, you can soak them ahead of time. Fill a bowl with enough water to cover the seeds or nuts and soak for at least 30 minutes, preferably overnight if time permits.

Nutritional analysis per serving (375 ml): calories 318, fat 26 g, saturated fat 3 g, cholesterol 0 mg, fiber 9 g, protein 8 g, carbohydrate 16 g, sodium 8 mg

THE CORE PLAN LUNCH RECIPES

Below are the instructions for creating your own salad bar, as well as five delicious soup recipes for you to choose from. Just a reminder: be sure to add 100 to 175 g of the protein of your choice – chicken, turkey, salmon, omega-3 eggs, tofu, or tempeh – either mixed into your soup or salad, or on the side.

Dr. Hyman's Super Salad Bar

Why go to a salad bar when you can create your own at home? To make this easy, start your week by setting up your own salad bar fixings.

Preparation:

■ Wash veggies, cut them into convenient salad-size bits, and store in sealed glass containers all in one location in your refrigerator. Cut enough for 2 to 3 days and repeat throughout the ten days as needed for freshness. Add different veggies at least twice a week for variety.

■ Make your salad the night before so you can grab- and-go on your way out the door. Store dressing in a separate container.

■ Store items not requiring refrigeration in small glass jars, preferably on a single shelf so they're easy to find. Toasted and raw nuts and seeds stay fresh for weeks when sealed in glass jars.

■ Ready, set, prep: Pick a variety of items from the list below and add them to your shopping list each week. Start by choosing your greens. Consider mixing various types of greens together— I like having some romaine with rocket to balance out texture. Avoid iceberg lettuce; it is hardly green and has almost no nutrients. Then choose your veggies, protein, healthy fats, and dressing. Select different options each day to keep your palate happy.

Greens (60 g per salad)

■ Rocket
■ Spinach
■ Mixed greens
■ Romaine lettuce

- Watercress
- Kale

Vegetables (125 to 250 g per salad, except as noted)

- Cucumber
- Peppers: red, green, yellow
- Sprouts: sunflower, pea shoots, clover, etc.
- Tomatoes: grape, cherry
- Carrots
- Beetroot (40 to 75 g)
- Red onions (40 to 75 g)
- Spring onions (40 to 75 g)
- Broccoli, lightly steamed
- Cauliflower, lightly steamed
- Cabbage: red, green, pak choi, etc.
- Mushrooms
- Sugarsnap peas
- Asparagus
- Artichoke hearts (packed in water in glass jars)
- Hearts of palm (packed in water in glass jars)
- Kalamata olives
- Courgettes
- Roasted aubergine
- Herbs, dried: parsley, basil, oregano, dill, coriander, mint, etc. (1 teaspoon)
- Herbs, fresh: mint, parsley, basil (25 g), dill, and oregano (25 g)

Protein (100 to 175 g)

- Canned fish (packed in water): salmon, sardines, herring, etc. (avoid tuna; it has too much mercury)
- Chicken (baked or roasted)
- Turkey (baked or roasted)
- Tofu
- Tempeh

- Hard-boiled eggs (2)
- Cooked prawns
- Leftover chicken or seafood from dinner

Healthy fats (choose one)

- Avocado (¼ to ½)
- Nuts, raw: almonds, cashews, walnuts, hazelnuts, Brazil nuts, pecans, etc. (70 g)
- Seeds, raw: flax, chia, hemp, sunflower, pumpkin, sesame, etc. (40 g)

Dressing (1 to 2 tablespoons per salad)

Here is the basic principle for making simple salad dressing. You can get creative with these ingredients; experiment and find out what you like.

Start by mixing oil with lemon (or lime) juice or vinegar, at a ratio of ¾ oil to ¼ lemon or vinegar (or 3 to 1 oil to vinegar).

- Oil: extra virgin olive, flax, walnut, or avocado oil
- Lemon or lime juice, or cider, balsamic, or wine vinegar
- Optional: Dijon mustard (mixed with lemon or vinegar)
- Optional: seasonings, including salt, freshly ground black pepper,
- fresh or dried herbs, such as basil, oregano, garlic, onion, and rosemary
- Optional (to make your dressing creamy): avocado or tahini (sesame paste)

The Core Plan Lunch Soups

CREAMY CAULIFLOWER SOUP

Serves: 4 Prep time: 15 minutes Cook time: 15 minutes

- 2 tablespoons extra virgin olive oil (reserve ¼ teaspoon for serving)
- ½ medium onion, diced
- 2 garlic cloves, sliced
- 1 medium cauliflower, cut into 5-cm chunks

- 35 g raw cashews
- 2 tablespoons sesame seeds or 1 tablespoon tahini paste
- ¼ avocado
- salt and freshly ground black pepper, to taste
- 1 tablespoon chopped fresh parsley

Heat the oil in a medium saucepan over a medium heat. Add the onion and garlic and sauté for 5 minutes, until translucent. Then add 1 litre water plus the cauliflower, cashews, and sesame seeds or tahini. Bring to the boil, reduce the heat to low, and simmer for 10 to 15 minutes, or until the cauliflower is tender. Let cool for 5 minutes. Purée the soup, then blend with the avocado until smooth. Season with salt and pepper. Drizzle with the reserved olive oil and the chopped parsley. Serve warm or chilled with your favorite salad and protein of your choice.

Nutritional analysis per serving (375 ml): calories 169, fat 12 g, saturated fat 2 g, cholesterol 0 mg, fiber 6 g, protein 6 g, carbohydrate 14 g, sodium 47 mg

CHICKEN SOUP FOR THE CAUSE

Serves: 4 Prep time: 15 to 20 minutes Cook time: 55 minutes

- 1 tablespoon extra virgin olive oil
- 1 small chicken, cut into quarters (remove the giblets; optional to remove skin)
- 3 medium carrots, peeled and sliced into half-moons
- 4 celery sticks, diced
- 2 medium onions, diced
- 1 litre reduced-sodium chicken stock
- salt and freshly ground black pepper, to taste
- 70 g kale or spinach
- 60 g fresh parsley, chopped

Heat the oil in a medium saucepan over a medium heat. Brown the chicken for 2 to 3 minutes on each side. Remove and set aside. Add the vegetables (minus the kale or spinach) to the pan and cook for 4 to 5 minutes. Put the chicken back into the pan, add the chicken stock, and bring to the boil. Reduce the heat to low, cover, and simmer for about

45 minutes, until the chicken starts to fall off the bones (you might want to add more liquid). Remove the bones. Skim any grease off the top with a ladle. Season with salt and pepper. Add the kale or spinach and allow them to wilt. Add the parsley and serve with a green salad.

Nutritional analysis per serving (450 ml): calories 246, fat 7 g, saturated fat 1 g, cholesterol 73 mg, fiber 4 g, protein 32 g, carbohydrate 13 g, sodium 291 mg

Courgette and Watercress Soup

Serves: 4 Prep time: 10 minutes Cook time: 20 minutes
- 2 tablespoons extra virgin olive oil (reserve ¼ teaspoon for serving)
- 1 medium onion, diced
- 4 celery sticks, diced
- 4 medium courgettes, diced
- 1 tablespoon almond butter or 70 g raw cashew nuts
- 1 litre reduced-sodium vegetable stock
- 275 g watercress, stems removed, chopped
- salt and freshly ground black pepper, to taste

In a medium saucepan, heat the oil over a medium heat. Add the onion and celery and cook for 5 minutes, until translucent. Add the courgettes and sauté for another 3 minutes. Add the almond butter or cashews and the vegetable stock and bring to the boil. Reduce the heat to low and simmer for 5 minutes, until the courgettes are tender. Add the watercress and cook for 3 more minutes, then turn off the heat. Using a slotted spoon, transfer the vegetables to a blender with about 250 ml stock and blend until smooth. Pour back into the pan and stir well. Season with salt and pepper. Drizzle each serving with some of the reserved olive oil and serve with a salad and protein of your choice.

Nutritional analysis per serving (450 ml): calories 225, fat 17 g, saturated fat 2 g, cholesterol 0 mg, fiber 5 g, protein 7 g, carbohydrate 17 g, sodium 180 mg

CREAMY ASPARAGUS SOUP

Serves: 6 Prep time: 10 minutes Cook time: 25 minutes

- 1 tablespoon extra virgin olive oil
- 3 garlic cloves, crushed
- 1 head cauliflower, cut into small florets
- 1 kg asparagus, trimmed and cut into 1-cm pieces
- ¼ teaspoon cayenne pepper
- 1.5 litres reduced-sodium vegetable or chicken stock, or water
- salt and freshly ground black pepper, to taste

In a medium saucepan, heat the oil over a medium–high heat. Add the garlic and cook for 1 minute. Add the cauliflower, asparagus, and cayenne pepper. Cook for 4 to 5 minutes, stirring frequently. Pour in the stock or water and bring the soup to the boil. Reduce the heat to low and simmer until the cauliflower is fully cooked, 5 to 8 minutes. Purée the soup until smooth, about 2 minutes. Season to taste with salt and black pepper. If the soup is too thick, thin it with a little more stock or water. If adding more liquid, return the soup to the hob, bring to a gentle simmer, and heat to the desired temperature. Serve with a salad and protein of your choice.

Nutritional analysis per serving (250 ml): calories 99, fat 4 g, saturated fat 0 g, cholesterol 0 mg, fiber 7 g, protein 6 g, carbohydrate 14 g, sodium 224 mg

GREEN GODDESS BROCCOLI AND ROCKET SOUP

Serves: 4 Prep time: 5 minutes Cook time: 20 minutes

- 1 teaspoon extra virgin olive oil
- ½ medium onion, chopped
- 2 garlic cloves, finely chopped
- 1 large head broccoli, cut into medium florets
- 1 handful rocket
- 625 ml low-sodium vegetable stock
- 120 ml unsweetened coconut milk
- juice of ½ lemon, or more if desired
- salt and freshly ground black pepper, to taste

Heat the olive oil in a medium saucepan over a medium-high heat. Add the onion and garlic and cook until soft, about 3 minutes. Add the broccoli and rocket. Stir frequently until the broccoli is bright green and the rocket has wilted, 4 to 5 minutes. Pour in the stock and bring the soup to the boil. Reduce the heat to low and simmer until the broccoli is fully cooked, 5 to 8 minutes. Purée the soup until smooth. Pour in the coconut milk and lemon juice and blend for another 30 seconds. Season with salt and pepper; add more lemon juice if desired. If the soup is too thick, thin it with a little more coconut milk or water and reheat to the desired temperature. Serve with a salad and protein of your choice.

Nutritional analysis per serving (300 ml): calories 104, fat 4 g, saturated fat 1 g, cholesterol 0 mg, fiber 5 g, protein 5 g, carbohydrate 13 g, sodium 289 mg

THE CORE PLAN DINNERS

GRIDDLED SALMON WITH ONION MARMALADE OVER GREENS

Serves: 4 Prep time: 20 minutes Cook time: 15 minutes

- 2 medium red onions, thinly sliced
- 2 tablespoons extra virgin olive oil, plus extra for brushing the salmon
- 1 tablespoon cider vinegar
- salt and freshly ground black pepper, to taste
- 4 salmon fillets (100 to 175 g each)
- 160 g rocket
- juice of ½ lemon, plus 1 lemon cut into 4 wedges
- 1 tablespoon chopped fresh parsley

Heat a griddle pan. In a bowl mix the onions, olive oil, vinegar, and salt and pepper. Place the onions in the middle of a large piece of foil; crimp it closed and place it in the pan. Heat for about 10 minutes, until the onions are soft, shaking the foil from time to time.

Cut each salmon fillet into 2 or 3 strips, brush with olive oil, and season with salt and pepper. Place each strip on the griddle pan and cook for 2 minutes on each side, or until cooked through. Let cool. Arrange the rocket on plates, sit the salmon on top and drizzle with lemon juice. Combine the chopped parsley with the onions and place a spoonful on top of each salad. Serve with a lemon wedge.

Nutritional analysis per serving (100 g salmon, 40 g rocket): calories 244, fat 17g, saturated fat 2 g, cholesterol 71 mg, fiber 2 g, protein 27 g, carbohydrate 8 g, sodium 312 mg

GRILLED SNAPPER WITH SALAD

Serves: 4 Prep time: 20 minutes Cook time: 6 minutes

- 4 snapper fillets (100 to 175 g each)
- 1 teaspoon extra virgin olive oil
- salt and freshly ground black pepper, to taste
- 1 lemon, cut into 4 wedges

SALAD:

- 1 head romaine lettuce, outer leaves removed
- 100 g rocket
- ½ avocado, diced
- 100g sprouts (see page 272)
- 6 radishes, cut in half and thinly sliced
- 150 g cherry tomatoes, halved
- 2 tablespoons freshly grated carrot
- 2 tablespoons freshly grated beetroot
- 2 tablespoons extra virgin olive oil
- juice of 1 lemon
- 1 tablespoon Dijon mustard

PREPARE THE SALAD

Chop the lettuce and rocket and combine in a bowl with the avocado, sprouts, radishes, tomatoes, carrot, and beetroot. In a separate bowl, whisk together the olive oil, lemon juice, and mustard. Pour the dressing over the salad. Divide among 4 plates and set aside.

PREPARE THE FISH

Heat the grill, or place a griddle pan over a medium heat. Brush each piece of fish with olive oil and season with salt and pepper. When the grill or griddle is hot, cook the fish for 3 minutes on each side, or until cooked through. Serve on top of the salad with a lemon wedge on the side.

Nutritional analysis per serving (100 g snapper, 100 g salad with dressing): calories 330, fat 17 g, saturated fat 2 g, cholesterol 53 mg, fiber 7 g, protein 34 g, carbohydrate 12 g, sodium 146 mg

ASIAN-FLAVORED CHICKEN SKEWERS

Serves: 4 Prep time: 35 to 60 minutes Cook time: 10 minutes

- 750 g boneless, skinless chicken breasts, cut into 1-cm strips

MARINADE:

- 120 ml low-sodium, gluten-free tamari
- 1 teaspoon grated fresh root ginger
- 3 garlic cloves, crushed
- 2 tablespoons sesame oil
- 1½ teaspoons five-spice powder

First, place 12 bamboo skewers in water and leave to soak for at least 20 minutes.

PREPARE THE MARINADE:

Combine all the marinade ingredients in a large, shallow baking dish.

PREPARE THE SKEWERS:

Thread the chicken onto the soaked skewers, leaving a 2-cm gap at each end. Place the skewers in the marinade dish, turning them to coat in the liquid. Cover and refrigerate for 30 to 60 minutes.

Heat the grill until very hot. Cook for 2 minutes on each side. Serve over a bed of Wilted Leafy Greens (see recipe below).

Nutritional analysis per serving (3 skewers): calories 225, fat 9 g, saturated fat 2 g, cholesterol 98 mg, fiber 0 g, protein 37 g, carbohydrate 1 g, sodium 137 mg

WILTED LEAFY GREENS

Serves: 4 Prep time: 10 minutes

- 275 g kale, stems removed
- 135 g watercress or 225 g spring greens, stems removed
- 250 g spinach
- 120 ml water
- 2 tablespoons extra virgin olive oil
- salt and freshly ground black pepper, to taste

Tear the greens into 5-cm pieces. Heat a large saucepan over a medium heat and add the water, olive oil, and kale. Cover and let the kale wilt for 1 to 2 minutes. Add the watercress or greens and allow them to wilt for another 1 to 2 minutes. Finally, add the spinach and let wilt for another 1 to 2 minutes. Drain off any excess water, add salt and pepper, and serve.

Nutritional analysis per serving (275 g): calories 128 , fat 8 g, saturated fat 0 g, cholesterol 0 mg, fiber 4 g, protein 6 g, carbohydrate 12 g, sodium 106 mg

HERB-CRUSTED CHICKEN BREASTS WITH ROASTED GARLIC

Serves: 4 Prep time: 20 minutes Cook time: 50 minutes

- 3 tablespoons extra virgin olive oil
- 2 heads garlic, tops cut off
- 4 boneless, skinless chicken breasts (100 to 175 g each)
- 1 tablespoon chopped fresh parsley
- 1 tablespoon chopped fresh rosemary
- 1 tablespoon chopped fresh thyme
- optional: ½ tablespoon chopped fresh sage
- ½ teaspoon sea salt
- freshly ground black pepper
- 35 g macadamia nuts or cashews, crushed
- 1 tablespoon Dijon mustard
- 1 bunch asparagus, trimmed
- 100 g salad greens

Preheat the oven to 190°C/Gas 5. Drizzle 1 tablespoon olive oil over the heads of garlic and roast in the oven for 30 to 40 minutes. Meanwhile, place each chicken breast in a plastic bag and pound firmly with a meat mallet or small saucepan to flatten slightly. Mix the herbs, salt, pepper and nuts in a small bowl and place the mixture on a flat plate. Brush each breast with a thin layer of Dijon mustard and coat each side with the herb mix.

Heat 1 tablespoon olive oil in a sauté pan over a medium heat. Sauté the breasts with the smooth, rounded side down for 3 to 4 minutes. Reduce the heat to low and turn over the breasts, cooking for another 3 minutes, until cooked through. Remove from the pan and set aside.

Heat 1 tablespoon olive oil in a clean pan over a medium heat. Sauté the asparagus for 3 to 4 minutes, until tender. Remove from the heat. Slice the chicken breasts on an angle. Squeeze the roasted garlic out of its skin and divide it evenly on top each serving of chicken. Arrange the asparagus over the greens.

Nutritional analysis per serving (100-g chicken breast, about 5 asparagus spears, and 25 g greens): calories 290, fat 16 g, saturated fat 3 g, cholesterol 65 mg, fiber 4 g, protein 28 g, carbohydrate 10 g, sodium 301 mg

BAKED COD WITH OLIVE AND CAPER PESTO

Serves: 4 Prep time: 15 minutes Cook time: 20 minutes
- 180 g stoned Kalamata olives
- 35 g capers, drained
- 1 tablespoon lemon zest, plus juice of 1 lemon
- 60 g fresh parsley, roughly chopped
- 2 garlic cloves
- 60 g raw walnuts
- 50 ml extra virgin olive oil
- 4 fillets of cod or other white fish (100 to 175 g each)

Preheat the oven to 180°C/Gas 4. In a food processor, combine the olives, capers, lemon zest and juice, parsley, garlic, and walnuts and process for 20 seconds. Drizzle in the olive oil while the motor is running; pulse to combine. Spread about 1 tablespoon of the olive and caper pesto onto each fish fillet. Place the fish in a greased ovenproof dish. Bake for 20 minutes and serve alongside Broccoli Rabe with Garlic and Cherry Tomatoes (see recipe below).

Nutritional analysis per serving (100g fish fillet with 1 tablespoon pesto): calories 390, fat 28 g, saturated fat 3 g, cholesterol 62 mg, fiber 3 g, protein 31 g, carbohydrate 6 g, sodium 647 mg

BROCCOLI RABE WITH GARLIC AND CHERRY TOMATOES

Serves: 4 Prep time: 5 minutes Cook time: 4 minutes
- 2 tablespoons extra virgin olive oil
- 4 garlic cloves, chopped
- 2 bunches broccoli rabe (rapini), trimmed
- 120 ml water
- 300 g cherry tomatoes, halved
- salt and freshly ground black pepper, to taste

Heat the olive oil in a large saucepan over a medium heat. Add the garlic and sauté for 10 seconds, then add the broccoli rabe and sauté until wilted slightly. Add the water and tomatoes, then cover and steam for 3 minutes, or until the greens are tender. Season with salt and pepper.

Nutritional analysis per serving (220 g): calories 116 , fat 8 g, saturated fat 0 g, cholesterol 0 mg, fiber 4 g, protein 4 g, carbohydrate 10 g, sodium 276 mg

ROAST CHICKEN BREAST WITH ROSEMARY

Serves: 4 Prep time: 10 minutes Cook time: 10 minutes
- 1 tablespoon finely chopped fresh rosemary
- 2 tablespoons Dijon mustard
- zest of 1 lemon
- 1 tablespoon olive oil
- 4 boneless, skinless chicken breasts (100 to 175 g each)
- salt and freshly ground black pepper, to taste

Preheat the oven to 200°C/Gas 6. Combine the chopped rosemary, mustard, lemon zest, and olive oil in a small bowl to make a paste and rub over both sides of each chicken breast. Season with salt and pepper and bake in a greased ovenproof baking dish for 5 minutes. Turn down the heat to 180°C/Gas 4 and cook for an additional 5 minutes or so; the chicken should be firm but not pink inside. Use a meat thermometer to ensure that the temperature is at least 74°C in the center. Be careful not to overcook. Serve with Baked Courgettes and Tomatoes (see recipe below).

Nutritional analysis per serving (100-g chicken breast): calories 145, fat 5 g, saturated fat 1 g, cholesterol 60 mg, fiber 2 g, protein 24 g, carbohydrate 5 g, sodium 138 mg

BAKED COURGETTES AND TOMATOES

Serves: 4 Prep time: 10 minutes Cook time: 10 minutes
- 2 tablespoons extra virgin olive oil, plus extra for greasing
- 4 courgettes, sliced on the diagonal into 5-mm pieces

- 4 tomatoes, sliced
- 2 onions, thinly sliced
- salt and freshly ground black pepper, to taste
- 1 avocado, stoned and diced
- 25 g fresh basil leaves

Preheat the oven to 190°C/Gas 5. Grease a baking tray with olive oil and arrange alternate slices of the courgettes, tomatoes, and onions, making 4 layers. Drizzle with the 2 tablespoons olive oil and season with salt and pepper. Bake for 10 minutes. Serve scattered with the diced avocado and the basil.

Nutritional analysis per serving (200 g vegetables, ¼ avocado):
calories 236, fat 15 g, saturated fat 2 g, cholesterol 0 mg, fiber 8 g, protein 5 g, carbohydrate 17 g, sodium 132 mg

STIR-FRIED VEGETABLES WITH ALMONDS

Serves: 4 Prep time: 20 minutes Cook time: 10 minutes

- 1 tablespoon extra virgin olive oil
- 1 tablespoon sesame oil
- 2 celery sticks, thinly sliced on the diagonal
- 1 onion, cut in half and thinly sliced
- 2 carrots, peeled and cut into half-moons
- 180 g broccoli florets or sliced pak choi
- 1 red or yellow pepper, seeded and sliced into strips
- optional: 450 g organic firm tofu, cubed
- 5-cm piece fresh root ginger, peeled and cut into matchsticks
- 2 garlic cloves, sliced
- 1 jalapeño chili, seeded and thinly sliced
- 6 mushrooms, stalks removed, thinly sliced
- 75 g whole raw almonds
- 50 ml water (more if needed)
- 2 tablespoons low-sodium, gluten-free tamari
- small handful basil leaves
- 3 spring onions, thinly sliced on the diagonal

In a large sauté pan or wok, heat the olive oil and sesame oil over a medium-high heat. Add the celery, onions, and carrots and stir-fry for 2 minutes. Add the broccoli or pak choi, peppers, and tofu, if using, and stir-fry another 2 minutes. Add the ginger, garlic, chili, and mushrooms and cook for 2 more minutes. Add the almonds, a little of the water as needed, and the tamari, and continue to stir-fry until the vegetables are cooked but still crunchy. Toss with the basil and spring onions just before serving.

Nutritional analysis per serving (150 g vegetables with 85 g tofu):
calories 271, fat 18 g, saturated fat 2 g, cholesterol 0 mg, fiber 6 g, protein 15 g, carbohydrate 18 g, sodium 408 mg

Nutritional analysis per serving (200 g vegetables without tofu):
calories 180, fat 15 g, saturated fat 1 g, cholesterol 0 mg, fiber 5 g, protein 6 g, carbohydrate 16g, sodium 342 mg

GRILLED PEPPER STEAK

Serves: 4 Prep time: 10 minutes Cook time: 7 to 8 minutes
- 4 pieces rump steak, or cut of your choice (150 g each)
- 1 tablespoon extra virgin olive oil
- 1 tablespoon freshly ground black pepper
- optional: 1 teaspoon ground chili pepper
- ½ teaspoon salt
- 1 tablespoon chopped fresh parsley

Heat the grill or a griddle pan. Brush each piece of steak with ¼ tablespoon of the olive oil. Combine the peppers and salt in a small bowl and rub the steaks with the mixture; let sit for 5 minutes. Grill or griddle the steaks for 3 to 4 minutes on each side (or until done to your liking). Let stand for 5 minutes before slicing. Sprinkle with chopped parsley and serve with salad of your choice.

Nutritional analysis per serving (150-g steak): calories 353, fat 22 g, saturated fat 7 g, cholesterol 78 mg, fiber 5 g, protein 41 g, carbohydrate 5 g, sodium 356 mg

Steamed Snapper with Ginger and Spring onions

Serves: 4 Prep time: 10 minutes Cook time: 10 minutes

- 4 snapper fillets, or fish of your choice (100 to 175 g each)
- 8 shiitake mushrooms, cut into quarters
- 2.5-cm piece fresh root ginger, peeled and thinly sliced
- 1 bunch asparagus, trimmed and sliced on the diagonal into 5-cm pieces
- 4 spring onions, sliced on the diagonal into 2.5-cm pieces
- 2 garlic cloves, sliced
- 2 tablespoons low-sodium, gluten-free tamari
- 475 ml fish stock or water
- 1 tablespoon sesame oil

Arrange the fish fillets in a 20-cm sauté pan. Add the mushrooms, ginger, asparagus, spring onions, garlic, tamari, and fish stock or water. Cover with a lid, place over a medium heat, and bring to the boil. Reduce the heat and simmer for about 7 minutes, until the fish is cooked through. Serve in individual bowls with the cooking stock, and drizzle with sesame oil.

Nutritional analysis per serving (100 g fish, with vegetables): calories 245, fat 5 g, saturated fat 1 g, cholesterol 0 mg, fiber 5 g, protein 27 g, carbohydrate 26 g, sodium 437 mg

Grilled Tofu with Coriander Pesto

Serves: 4 Prep time: 20 minutes Cook time: 10 minutes

- 3 tablespoons low-sodium, gluten-free tamari
- 2 tablespoons sesame oil
- 450 g organic firm tofu, cut into 8 slices
- 2 courgettes, sliced on the diagonal into 5-mm pieces

PESTO:

- 75 g fresh basil, stems removed
- 35 g fresh coriander, stems removed
- 2 garlic cloves, chopped
- 1-cm piece fresh root ginger, peeled and chopped

- 3 spring onions, trimmed and roughly chopped
- 35 g pine nuts or raw walnuts
- 120 ml extra virgin olive oil (reserve 1 tablespoon for serving)
- 100 g rocket or other favorite greens
- salt and freshly ground black pepper, to taste

Heat the grill or a griddle pan. In a large bowl, combine the tamari and sesame oil; add the tofu and courgette slices and marinate for 10 minutes.

Grill or griddle the courgettes first, about 2 minutes on each side, then grill or griddle the tofu for about 3 minutes on each side. Set aside.

PREPARE THE PESTO:

Place all the ingredients except the rocket or other greens, the salt and pepper, and the reserved olive oil in a food processor and pulse until smooth. If necessary, add 2 tablespoons of water for a thinner consistency. Season with salt and pepper.

ASSEMBLE THE DISH:

Lightly toss the rocket or other greens with the reserved olive oil; divide among 4 plates, placing the piles on one side. Arrange the tofu and courgettes on the other side of the plates and drizzle with the pesto.

Nutritional analysis per serving (2 pieces tofu, ¼ courgette, 2 tablespoons pesto): calories 456, fat 42 g, saturated fat 6 g, cholesterol 0 mg, fiber 5 g, protein 16 g, carbohydrate 12 g, sodium 562 mg

ADVENTURE PLAN LUNCH OPTIONS

KALE AND RED CABBAGE SLAW WITH TURKEY MEATBALLS

Serves: 4 Prep time: 20 minutes Cook time: 20 minutes

KALE AND CABBAGE SLAW:

- 2 bunches kale, stalks removed, thinly sliced
- ½ head red cabbage, thinly sliced
- 35 g raw sunflower seeds
- 2 tablespoons extra virgin olive oil
- juice of ½ lemon
- ¼ teaspoon salt
- optional: 1 avocado, stoned and sliced

TURKEY MEATBALLS:

- 450 g minced turkey
- ½ onion, finely diced
- 25 g celery, finely diced
- 1 tablespoon tomato purée (plus extra for topping)
- 1 egg
- 1 teaspoon dried thyme
- 1 teaspoon dried sage
- 1 teaspoon dried rosemary
- ½ teaspoon salt
- ½ teaspoon freshly ground black pepper

PREPARE THE SLAW:

Combine the slaw ingredients in a bowl, then divide equally between 4 plates. If desired, garnish with ¼ avocado per portion.

Preheat the oven to 180°C/Gas 4. In a large bowl, combine all the meatball ingredients, except the extra tomato purée for topping. Using an ice cream scoop or your hands, form the mixture into balls the size of a golf ball and place on a baking tray (the recipe should yield 12 to 16 balls). Top each meatball with 1 teaspoon extra tomato purée. Bake for 20 minutes, turning once. Serve alongside the slaw.

Nutritional analysis per serving (4 meatballs with 180 g slaw):
calories 322, fat 18 g, saturated fat 4 g, cholesterol 106 mg, fiber 5 g, protein 29 g, carbohydrate 17 g, sodium 462 mg

Pak Choi Salad with Tofu or Raw Almonds

Serves: 4 Prep time: 30 minutes

- 2 medium heads pak choi, thinly sliced
- 40 g wakame, covered with just enough water to soften
- 2 tablespoons white sesame seeds
- 135 g asparagus, trimmed and thinly sliced on the diagonal
- 2 celery sticks, thinly sliced
- 1 small carrot, peeled and thinly sliced on the diagonal
- 4 spring onions, thinly sliced on the diagonal
- 4 medium red radishes, thinly sliced
- 2 tablespoons grated fresh root ginger
- 1 tablespoon roughly chopped coriander
- 2 tablespoons cider vinegar
- juice of 2 limes, plus zest of 1 lime
- 4 tablespoons low-sodium, gluten-free tamari
- ½ teaspoon cayenne pepper
- 1 avocado, stoned and cubed
- 450 g firm tofu, cubed, or 150 g raw whole almonds

Toss all the ingredients together in a large bowl. For maximum flavor, allow the salad to sit for 30 minutes before serving.

Nutritional analysis per serving (75 g salad with tofu): calories 252, fat 14 g, saturated fat 2 g, cholesterol 0 mg, fiber 7 g, protein 15 g, carbohydrate 20 g, sodium 444 mg

Nutritional analysis per serving (75 g salad with almonds): calories 227, fat 4 g, saturated fat 1 g, cholesterol 0 mg, fiber 6 g, protein 10 g, carbohydrate 19 g, sodium 432 mg

WALNUT PÂTÉ WITH FRESH TOMATO SALSA

Serves: 4 Prep time: 20 minutes

- 200 g raw walnuts
- 4 celery sticks, diced
- ½ red onion, finely diced
- 1 tablespoon chopped fresh parsley
- 1 teaspoon fresh thyme
- 1 tablespoon lemon zest
- 1 tablespoon extra virgin olive oil
- 1 teaspoon freshly ground black pepper
- ¼ teaspoon salt
- 4 romaine lettuce leaves, to serve

TOMATO SALSA:

- 3 ripe tomatoes, seeded and diced
- juice of 1 lime
- 1 tablespoon chopped coriander
- ½ red onion, diced
- ¼ teaspoon cayenne pepper or ½ jalapeño chili pepper, seeded and finely chopped
- ½ teaspoon cumin
- ½ teaspoon salt
- ½ teaspoon freshly ground black pepper

Place the walnuts in a food processor and pulse for 20 seconds. Add the celery and onion and pulse again for 20 seconds. Add all the other ingredients, except the lettuce, and pulse for another 10 seconds. Transfer the pâté to a bowl.

PREPARE THE SALSA:

Toss all the ingredients together in a medium bowl. Taste and add more cayenne or chili as desired.

ASSEMBLE THE DISH:

Serve the pâté on the lettuce leaves and top with the salsa.

Nutritional analysis per serving (180 g pâté with 2 tablespoons salsa): calories 406, fat 36 g, saturated fat 2 g, cholesterol 0 mg, fiber 6 g, protein 15 g, carbohydrate 14 g, sodium 324 mg

VEGETABLE ROLLS WITH SHREDDED CHICKEN AND NUT CREAM

Serves: 4 Prep time: 30 minutes Cook time: 10 minutes

VEGETABLE MIXTURE:

- 1 medium carrot, peeled and thinly sliced or shredded
- 3 medium courgettes, thinly sliced or shredded
- ½ head white cabbage, shredded
- ¼ head red cabbage, shredded
- handful fresh mint leaves, cut into strips
- 50 g spring onions, sliced on the diagonal

POACHED CHICKEN BREASTS:

- 1 litre water
- 1 sprig fresh thyme
- 1 sprig fresh rosemary
- 1 teaspoon salt
- 4 boneless, skinless chicken breasts (100 to 175 g each)

NUT CREAM:

- 135 g pine nuts or raw cashews
- 120 ml fresh lemon juice
- pinch of salt
- optional: ¼ teaspoon cayenne pepper

SPRING GREEN WRAPS:

- 4 spring green leaves, stems removed, halved lengthways
- 500 ml boiling water

PREPARE THE VEGETABLE MIXTURE:

Combine all the ingredients in a large bowl.

PREPARE THE CHICKEN:

In a large saucepan, bring the water to the boil. Add the thyme, rosemary, and salt. Turn the heat down to a simmer and carefully add the chicken breasts. Cover and simmer for about 10 minutes; remove from the heat and let rest, covered, for about 10 minutes. When the breasts are cool, shred with a fork or by hand.

PREPARE THE NUT CREAM:

Place all the ingredients in a blender and blend until smooth but thick, adding water if needed.

ASSEMBLE THE ROLLS:

Lay the spring green leaves in a baking tin and slowly pour the boiling water over them so they soften; drain, let cool, and pat dry. Combine the nut cream, shredded chicken, and vegetable mixture. Lay one spring green leaf smooth side down and spoon about 50 g of filling onto one end. Roll up tightly. Continue until all the rolls are made and serve two per person.

Nutritional analysis per serving (2 spring green wraps with 1½ tablespoons nut cream per wrap): calories 455, fat 26 g, saturated fat 3 g, cholesterol 82 mg, fiber 9 g, protein 43 g, carbohydrate 21 g, sodium 504 mg

Chopped Vegetable Salad with Salmon

Serves: 4 Prep time: 15 minutes Cook time: 10 minutes

SALMON:

- 4 salmon fillets (100 to 175 g each)
- 1 tablespoon extra virgin olive oil
- salt and freshly ground black pepper, to taste

DRESSING:

- juice of ½ lemon
- 3 tablespoons extra virgin olive oil
- 1 teaspoon Dijon mustard

SALAD:

- 1 head romaine lettuce, outer leaves and core removed, cut into 4-cm pieces
- 1 cucumber, peeled, seeded, and diced
- ½ small red onion, diced
- 6 radishes, trimmed and diced
- 2 medium tomatoes, halved and seeded
- 1 yellow pepper, seeded and diced
- 1 tablespoon chopped fresh parsley
- small handful fresh basil leaves
- 1 tablespoon chopped fresh dill
- 1 heaped tablespoon drained capers, or stoned Kalamata olives, rinsed and cut in half

PREPARE THE SALMON:

Heat the grill or a griddle pan. Brush the salmon lightly with olive oil and season with salt and pepper. Grill or griddle for 3 minutes on each side, until firm to the touch or cooked through. When cool, break the salmon up with a fork.

PREPARE THE DRESSING:

In a small bowl, whisk together the lemon juice, olive oil, and mustard.

PREPARE THE SALAD:

Combine all the ingredients in a large bowl and add the salmon. Toss with the dressing and serve.

Nutritional analysis per serving (100 g salad, 100g salmon): calories 347, fat 21 g, saturated fat 3 g, cholesterol 70 mg, fiber 4 g, protein 27 g, carbohydrate 14 g, sodium 494 mg

Cucumber Salad with Sunflower Mock Tuna

Serves: 4 Prep time: 30 minutes

- 145 g raw almonds
- 275 g raw sunflower seeds
- 2 courgettes, peeled and cut into 2.5-cm cubes
- 2 tablespoons chopped red onion
- 25 g celery, chopped
- 1 tablespoon grated fresh root ginger
- 50 ml lemon juice
- 1 tablespoon low-sodium, gluten-free tamari
- 1 tablespoon finely chopped coriander
- 1 tablespoon finely chopped parsley
- optional: pinch of cayenne pepper
- salt and freshly ground black pepper, to taste
- optional: dulse flakes or thinly sliced nori

CUCUMBER AND TOMATO SALAD:

- 550 to 725 g fresh organic tomatoes, quartered or cut into chunks
- 2 medium cucumbers, seeded and diced
- 2 tablespoons extra virgin olive oil
- juice and zest of 1 lemon
- small handful fresh basil, sliced

PREPARE THE MOCK TUNA:

Place the almonds in a food processor and pulse for 30 seconds. Add the sunflower seeds and pulse again for 20 seconds. Add the courgettes, onions, and celery and pulse for another 20 seconds (until everything looks rice-size). Pour into a bowl and add the ginger, lemon juice, tamari, and fresh herbs. Add cayenne for desired heat. Mix well and season with the salt and pepper. Sprinkle with dulse flakes or thinly sliced nori, if using.

PREPARE THE SALAD:

Toss all the ingredients together in a bowl and serve alongside the mock tuna (on a bed of greens, if you like).

Nutritional analysis per serving (100 g mock tuna, 100 g cucumber salad): calories 405, fat 32 g, saturated fat 3 g, cholesterol 0 mg, fiber 9 g, protein 14 g, carbohydrate 26 g, sodium 326 mg

COD CAKES OVER MIXED GREENS

Serves: 4 Prep time: 20 minutes Cook time: 15 minutes

COD CAKES:

- 4 cod fillets (100 to 175 g each)
- 75 g pumpkin seeds or macadamia nuts
- 1 egg
- 1 tablespoon chopped fresh thyme
- 1 tablespoon chopped fresh parsley
- 50 g red onion, diced
- 1 tablespoon lemon zest, plus 1 teaspoon lemon juice
- 1 teaspoon Dijon mustard
- pinch of cayenne pepper
- ½ teaspoon salt
- ½ teaspoon freshly ground black pepper
- 1 tablespoon extra virgin olive oil

SALAD:

- 400 g mixed salad greens of your choice
- 2 medium tomatoes, cut into wedges
- 1 tablespoon extra virgin olive oil
- 1 tablespoon lemon juice

PREPARE THE FISH:

Put about 5mm water into a steamer or saucepan and bring to the boil. Add the cod fillets, cover, and cook over a medium heat for about 7 minutes, or until translucent. Let cool. Using a fork, break up the fish into flakes.

In a spice grinder or food processor, whiz the pumpkin seeds or macadamia nuts to the size of medium breadcrumbs. Alternatively, place the nuts in a plastic bag and crush with a rolling pin. In a large bowl, whisk the egg and add the herbs, onion, lemon zest, and juice. Add the fish flakes, mustard, cayenne, salt, and pepper. Form into 4 patties. Spread the ground seeds or nuts on a plate and coat the patties on all sides.

Heat the olive oil in a sauté pan over a medium heat. Cook the cod cakes for 3 minutes on each side.

ASSEMBLE THE DISH:

Serve each cod cake alongside or on top of the salad greens, garnish with tomato wedges, and drizzle with olive oil and lemon juice.

Nutritional analysis per serving (1 cod cake with salad): calories 322, fat 17 g, saturated fat 3 g, cholesterol 103 mg, fiber 3 g, protein 33 g, carbohydrate 10 g, sodium 482 mg

ROCKET, AVOCADO, AND GRILLED SNAPPER

Serves: 4 Prep time: 20 minutes Cook time: 7 minutes

FISH:

- 4 snapper fillets (100 g each)
- 1 tablespoon extra virgin olive oil
- salt and freshly ground black pepper, to taste
- 4 lemon wedges, for garnish

SALAD:

- 100 g rocket, large stems removed
- 1 head romaine lettuce, outer leaves and core removed
- ½ avocado, stoned and diced
- 100 g sprouts (see page 272)
- 6 red radishes, halved
- 175 g cherry tomatoes, halved
- 1 tablespoon freshly grated carrot
- 1 tablespoon freshly grated beetroot

DRESSING:

- 3 tablespoons extra virgin olive oil
- juice of 1 lemon
- 1 tablespoon Dijon mustard
- freshly ground black pepper, to taste

PREPARE THE FISH:

Heat the grill until hot or place a griddle pan over a medium heat. Brush each fish fillet with olive oil. Grill or griddle the fish for 3 minutes on each side. When the fish is cooked through, remove from the heat and season with salt and pepper.

PREPARE THE SALAD AND DRESSING:

Combine the salad ingredients in a bowl. In a separate small bowl, whisk the dressing ingredients together. Drizzle over the salad and toss. Divide the tossed salad among 4 plates.

ASSEMBLE THE DISH:

Place a fish fillet on top of each portion of salad and garnish with a wedge of lemon.

Nutritional analysis per serving (150 g salad, 100 g fish): calories 268, fat 16 g, saturated fat 2 g, cholesterol 58 mg, fiber 4 g, protein 25 g, carbohydrate 8 g, sodium 305 mg

SPICED TURKEY WRAP WITH WATERCRESS AND AVOCADO

Serves: 4 Prep time: 10 minutes Cook time: 20 minutes

SPICED TURKEY:

- 250 ml extra virgin olive oil
- 2 medium onions, thinly sliced
- 8 garlic cloves, crushed
- 5- to 10-cm piece fresh root ginger (depending on the degree of spice you like), peeled and grated
- 4 medium carrots, peeled and shredded
- 1 tablespoon cayenne pepper
- 4 teaspoons ground coriander
- 4 teaspoons ground turmeric
- ½ tablespoon ground cinnamon
- salt and freshly ground black pepper, to taste
- 550 g lean minced turkey
- 120 ml low-sodium chicken stock
- 1 tablespoon finely chopped fresh coriander

WRAPS:

- 16 large romaine leaves
- 2 avocados, stoned and mashed
- 60 g baby spinach
- 60 g watercress
- 1 lime, cut into wedges

PREPARE THE SPICED TURKEY:

Heat the oil in a wok or large heavy-based frying pan over a medium-high heat. Sauté the onions, garlic, and ginger, stirring constantly, until aromatic and softened, 3 to 4 minutes. Add the carrots, cayenne, ground coriander, turmeric, and cinnamon. Season to taste with salt and pepper and mix well. After a minute, add the turkey, using a fork or wooden spoon to crumble it into separate pieces. Gently stir the mixture together until the turkey is browned and cooked through, 6 to 8 minutes. Pour in the chicken stock and stir, scraping the bottom of the pan to release any tasty browned bits. Turn off the heat and fold in the fresh coriander. Transfer the turkey mixture to a small bowl.

ASSEMBLE THE DISH:

Lay the lettuce leaves out on a plate and spread a heaped teaspoon of the mashed avocado on each leaf. Add some spinach and watercress to each wrap. Top with small piles of the spiced turkey and roll up. Serve with the lime wedges on the side.

Nutritional analysis per serving (4 wraps): calories 566, fat 36 g, saturated fat 5 g, cholesterol 70 mg, fiber 9 g, protein 40 g, carbohydrate 27 g, sodium 314 mg

WATERCRESS AND ROCKET SALAD WITH POACHED EGGS

Serves: 4 Prep time: 10 minutes Cook time: 10 minutes

SALAD:

- 80 g rocket
- 80 g watercress
- 175 g cherry tomatoes, halved
- ½ cucumber, thinly sliced
- ½ avocado, stoned and chopped or sliced

DRESSING:

- 2 tablespoons extra virgin olive oil
- ½ teaspoon salt
- 1 teaspoon freshly ground black pepper
- juice of 1 lemon

EGGS:

- 8 omega-3 eggs
- optional: freshly ground black pepper or cayenne pepper

PREPARE THE SALAD AND DRESSING:

Toss the rocket, watercress, tomatoes, cucumbers, and avocado together in a bowl. In a separate bowl, whisk together the olive oil, salt, pepper, and lemon juice. Drizzle over the salad and toss. Divide the tossed salad among 4 plates.

PREPARE THE EGGS:

Add 2.5 cm water and ½ teaspoon of salt to a 25-cm saucepan. Bring to the boil, then lower the heat and keep at a simmer. Break 2 eggs into a small bowl. Carefully pour them into the hot water and repeat until all the eggs are in the saucepan. Cover and poach for about 3 minutes.

ASSEMBLE THE DISH:

Using a slotted spoon, remove the eggs from the water and place directly on the salad. Sprinkle with black pepper (or cayenne if you like things spicy hot).

Nutritional analysis per serving (150g salad, 2 eggs): calories 263, fat 19 g, saturated fat 4 g, cholesterol 350 mg, fiber 3 g, protein 14 g, carbohydrate 6 g, sodium 389 mg

ADVENTURE PLAN DINNERS

COCONUT CURRY WITH FISH OR TOFU

Serves: 4 Prep time: 20 minutes Cook time: 40 minutes

COCONUT CURRY:

- 3 tablespoons extra virgin coconut butter
- 1 teaspoon mustard seeds
- 1 teaspoon fenugreek seeds
- 1 to 2 fresh chilies, thinly sliced
- 2.5-cm piece fresh root ginger, peeled and coarsely chopped

- 2 garlic cloves, crushed
- optional: 6 curry leaves
- 2 medium onions, coarsely diced
- ½ teaspoon chili powder
- ½ teaspoon ground turmeric
- 6 medium tomatoes, seeded and coarsely chopped, or 400-g can low-sodium chopped tomatoes
- 1 litre low-sodium vegetable stock
- 120 ml unsweetened coconut milk
- salt, to taste

FISH OR TOFU:

- 4 cod fillets (100 g each), or 400 g firm tofu cut into 4 equal pieces

VEGETABLES:

- 100 g cauliflower florets
- 100 g sliced courgettes
- 70 g chopped baby pak choi
- 30 g spinach

GARNISH:

- 75 g chopped raw almonds or raw cashews
- handful fresh coriander, stems removed

PREPARE THE CURRY SAUCE:

In a large saucepan, heat 2 tablespoons of the coconut butter over a medium heat. Add the mustard seeds and reduce the heat to low. When the seeds start to pop, add the fenugreek, chilies, ginger, garlic, and curry leaves, if using. Stir for about 3 minutes, then add the diced onions and cook 5 minutes, until they are soft and slightly brown. Add the chili powder, turmeric, chopped tomatoes, and vegetable stock and bring to the boil. Reduce the heat and simmer for 15 minutes. Add the coconut milk and simmer for an additional 5 minutes. Season with salt and stir in the remaining coconut butter just before serving.

PREPARE THE FISH OR TOFU:

If using fish, add it to the sauce and cook for an additional 5 to 7 minutes, or until the fish is opaque inside. If using tofu, simmer for another 5 minutes.

PREPARE THE VEGETABLES:

Bring 120 ml water to the boil in a saucepan or sauté pan. If you are using a saucepan, place the vegetables in a metal or bamboo steamer inside the pan and cover with a lid. Steam for 3 to 5 minutes, until the vegetables are soft. If using a sauté pan, place the vegetables in the pan and cover. Turn the heat down to medium and let the vegetables simmer for 3 to 5 minutes.

ASSEMBLE THE DISH:

Divide the vegetables equally among 4 plates and serve the curry on top. Garnish with the almonds or cashews and fresh coriander.

Nutritional analysis per serving (250 ml curry sauce, 100 g vegetable medley, and 100 g fish): calories 463, fat 25 g, saturated fat 16 g, cholesterol 62 mg, fiber 9 g, protein 25 g, carbohydrate 28 g, sodium 207 mg

Nutritional analysis per serving (250 ml curry sauce, 100 g vegetable medley, and 100 g tofu): calories 423, fat 29 g, saturated fat 17 g, cholesterol 0 mg, fiber 10 g, protein 19 g, carbohydrate 30 g, sodium 129 mg

CHICKEN BREAST WITH RATATOUILLE AND STEAMED BROCCOLI

Serves: 4 Prep time: 35 minutes Cook time: 55 minutes

CHICKEN:

- 1 tablespoon extra virgin olive oil
- 3 garlic cloves, chopped
- 1 tablespoon chopped fresh thyme
- 1 tablespoon chopped fresh parsley
- 4 boneless, skinless chicken breasts (100 to 175 g each)

RATATOUILLE:

- 1 small aubergine, cut into 1-cm pieces (peeling is optional)
- 1 teaspoon salt
- 4 tablespoons extra virgin olive oil
- 2 courgettes, diced into 1-cm pieces
- 2 red peppers, seeded and cut into 1-cm pieces
- 2 medium onions, cut into 1-cm pieces
- 4 garlic cloves, finely chopped
- 400-g can low-sodium chopped tomatoes
- optional: 250 ml low-sodium vegetable stock
- 1 tablespoon chopped parsley
- 1 teaspoon finely chopped fresh thyme
- salt and freshly ground black pepper, to taste

BROCCOLI:

- 2 medium heads broccoli, cut into florets

PREPARE THE CHICKEN:

Combine the olive oil, garlic, thyme, and parsley in a large bowl, and add the chicken. Marinate for at least 15 minutes. Heat a griddle or heavy-based frying pan over a medium-high heat for 1 minute. Turn the heat down to medium and brown the chicken for 2 minutes on each side, or until golden brown.

PREPARE THE RATATOUILLE:

Sprinkle the aubergine with salt and place in a colander. Set aside for 10 minutes. After the aubergine has released its moisture, rinse it with water and pat dry. Heat 2 tablespoons of the olive oil in a 20-cm saucepan over a medium heat. When the oil is shimmering, add the aubergine to the pan. Cook lightly for 5 minutes, until it browns slightly. Set aside on a plate. Add 1 tablespoon olive oil and the courgettes to the empty pan and cook for 3 minutes, until slightly browned. Remove from the pan, and set aside. Add the red peppers and sauté for 5 minutes, until they soften. Remove from the pan and set aside. Add 1 tablespoon of the remaining olive oil, sauté the onions for 5 minutes until softened, then add the garlic and cook for 2 more minutes. Add the tomatoes and cook for another 5 minutes. Return the aubergine, courgettes, and peppers to the pan and simmer for 20 minutes. Add the stock (if you prefer a thinner consistency), then the parsley and thyme. Season with salt and pepper, and simmer for another 10 minutes. Meanwhile, continue with the next step.

PREPARE THE BROCCOLI:

Boil approximately 2.5 cm water in a saucepan. Add the broccoli, cover the pan, and steam for about 3 minutes, until just tender, but not soft. Drain well.

ASSEMBLE THE DISH:

Divide the ratatouille among 4 plates. Cut each chicken breast into 3 slices and place each breast on top of a plate of ratatouille. Serve with the broccoli on the side.

Nutritional analysis per serving (175 g chicken, 250 g ratatouille, and 150 g broccoli): calories 418, fat 18 g, saturated fat 3 g, cholesterol 66 mg, fiber 16 g, protein 39 g, carbohydrate 38 g, sodium 377 mg

GRILLED SALMON OR TOFU VEGETABLE KEBABS

Serves: 4 Prep time: 40 minutes Cook time: 10 minutes
- 1 onion, cut into large chunks
- 1 red or yellow pepper, seeded and cut into 2.5-cm chunks
- 12 button or chestnut mushrooms, stems removed
- 1 courgette, sliced into half-moons
- 450 g salmon or tofu (cut the tofu into 2.5-cm cubes)
- 50 ml extra virgin olive oil
- 1 tablespoon chopped fresh thyme
- 2 garlic cloves, crushed
- 65 g almond butter
- 1 tablespoon cider vinegar
- ½ chili pepper, seeded

- 2 tablespoons lime juice
- 250 ml water
- salt and freshly ground black pepper, to taste

Place 4 bamboo skewers in water and leave to soak for at least 20 minutes.

Thread the vegetables and fish or tofu alternately onto each skewer, pushing the pieces together firmly and leaving a 2-cm gap at each end. Combine the olive oil, thyme, and garlic in a large baking dish and add the skewers; marinate for 30 minutes or more.

Heat the grill or a griddle pan; while waiting, combine the almond butter, vinegar, chili, lime juice, and water in a blender and blend until smooth (add more chili if desired). Drain the kebabs and season them with salt and pepper. Cook salmon kebabs under the grill or in the griddle pan for 7 to 10 minutes, depending on the thickness of the fish. Cook tofu kebabs for 3 to 5 minutes on each side, until done. Serve with Sautéed Spring Greens (see recipe below).

Nutritional analysis per serving (1 skewer with salmon): calories 308, fat 18 g, saturated fat 2 g, cholesterol 45 mg, fiber 3 g, protein 27 g, carbohydrate 12 g, sodium 104 mg

Nutritional analysis per serving (1 skewer with tofu): calories 279, fat 20 g, saturated fat 3 g, cholesterol 0 mg, fiber 4 g, protein 15 g, carbohydrate 14 g, sodium 23 mg

Sautéed Spring Greens

Serves: 4 Prep time: 7 minutes Cook time: 7 minutes

- 2 bunches spring greens, stems removed
- 2 garlic cloves, thinly sliced lengthways
- 1 tablespoon extra virgin olive oil
- salt and freshly ground black pepper, to taste

Stack the greens together, roll them up, then slice thinly. Heat a sauté pan over a medium heat, add the olive oil and garlic, and cook for 30 seconds. Add the greens and cook until they are wilted and soft, about 7 minutes. Season with salt and pepper.

Nutritional analysis per serving (190 g greens): calories 67, fat 5 g, saturated fat 0 g, cholesterol 2 mg, fiber 1 g, protein 1 g, carbohydrate 5 g, sodium 43 mg

ROAST FISH CASSEROLE WITH FENNEL AND LEEKS

Serves: 4 Prep time: 20 minutes Cook time: 40 minutes

FISH:

- 2 tablespoons extra virgin olive oil
- 4 sea bass or cod fillets (100 to 175 g each)
- salt and freshly ground black pepper, to taste
- 2 medium fennel bulbs, trimmed and thinly sliced
- 2 leeks, white parts only, sliced
- 2 garlic cloves, crushed
- 475 ml low-sodium vegetable stock
- 4 medium tomatoes, diced
- 6 sprigs thyme or 6 lemon slices (reserve 4 for garnish)
- 2 tablespoons chopped fresh parsley
- 90 g stoned Kalamata olives, halved and rinsed

SPINACH:

- 350 g fresh spinach

PREPARE THE CASSEROLE:

Preheat the oven to 180°C/Gas 4. Heat an flameproof 20-cm casserole dish over a medium heat and add 1 tablespoon of the olive oil. Season the fish with salt and pepper and place in the pan. Brown each piece for about 2 minutes on each side. Remove from the pan and set aside.

Add the remaining olive oil to the empty casserole dish. Add the fennel, leeks, and garlic and cook over a low heat for 5 minutes. Add the stock and tomatoes and cook for another 5 minutes. Carefully return the fish to the pan and add 2 of the thyme sprigs or lemon slices, the parsley, and the olives. Cover and cook in the oven for 20 minutes.

While the fish is cooking, heat 50 ml water in a saucepan over a medium heat. Add the spinach, cover and cook for about 2 minutes. Drain in a colander and divide among 4 bowls.

Carefully remove the casserole from the oven. Using a slotted spoon, place the fish fillets on top of the spinach in each bowl and spoon the vegetables and the broth over the top. Garnish with sprigs of fresh thyme or slices of lemon if you prefer.

Nutritional analysis per serving (100 g fish, 225 g greens): calories 340, fat 16 g, saturated fat 2 g, cholesterol 62 mg, fiber 8 g, protein 31 g, carbohydrate 21 g, sodium 472 mg

ALMOND-FLAX CRUSTED CHICKEN

Serves: 4 Prep time: 35 minutes Cook time: 20 to 30 minutes

- 4 boneless, skinless chicken breasts (100 to 175 g each)
- 1 tablespoon extra virgin olive oil
- 1 tablespoon almond butter
- 1 teaspoon lemon juice
- 1 teaspoon salt
- pinch of cayenne pepper
- 1 teaspoon chopped fresh parsley
- 1 teaspoon paprika
- ⅓ teaspoon onion powder
- 3 tablespoons ground flaxseed
- 50 g ground almonds

Preheat the oven to 180°C/Gas 4. Rinse the chicken and pat dry with kitchen paper. Place the chicken breasts between sheets of cling film and pound with a meat mallet or small saucepan until thin. In a small bowl or food processor, combine the olive oil, almond butter, lemon juice, and all the seasoning. Spread the mixture on the chicken breasts and, if you have time, allow to sit for 10 to 15 minutes to enhance the flavor. Even better is to cover the chicken and leave it in the refrigerator for up to 24 hours before cooking.

Combine the flaxseed and ground almonds in a small bowl and set aside. Place the chicken breasts on a lightly oiled baking tray. Sprinkle half the almond-flax mixture evenly over one side of each chicken breast. Pat each chicken piece with your hand to make the "crust" stick to the chicken. Carefully turn over each chicken piece and repeat the process, using the remaining half of the almond-flax mixture. Place the chicken in the center of the oven and bake for 20 to 30 minutes, until the juices run clear, or a meat thermometer stuck in the thickest part registers 74°C.

Nutritional analysis per serving (100-g chicken breast): calories 262, fat 15 g, saturated fat 2 g, cholesterol 62 mg, fiber 4 g, protein 30 g, carbohydrate 4 g, sodium 325 mg

BEEF WITH PAK CHOI

Serves: 4 Prep time: 35 minutes Cook time: 20 minutes

- 3 tablespoons extra virgin olive oil
- 2 garlic cloves, thinly sliced
- 1 teaspoon freshly ground black pepper
- 2 tablespoons finely chopped fresh rosemary
- 1 tablespoon Dijon mustard
- salt, to taste
- 750 g flank steak, cut into 4 equal portions

VEGETABLES:

- 4 carrots, peeled and quartered
- 560 g pak choi, sliced into 5-mm pieces

SAUCE:

- 120 ml low-sodium beef stock
- 1 tablespoon low-sodium, gluten-free tamari

PREPARE THE STEAK:

Combine the olive oil, garlic, pepper, 1 tablespoon of the rosemary, and the mustard and rub the mixture over each piece of steak. Let rest for about 30 minutes. Season with salt. Heat the grill or a griddle pan until very hot. Lower the heat to medium, then sear each piece of steak to your desired degree of doneness; for medium-rare, this would be about 3 minutes per side. Remove the meat from the pan and allow to rest for a few minutes, then slice each steak into 4 equal pieces.

PREPARE THE VEGETABLES:

Place about 2.5 cm water in a 20-cm saucepan and bring to the boil over a medium heat. Add the carrots and steam, covered, for about 5 minutes. Add the pak choi and steam for 2 to 3 minutes, until all the vegetables are tender to the point of a knife.

PREPARE THE SAUCE:

Add the beef stock and tamari to the meat pan. Bring to the boil, scraping up all the browned bits, then lower the heat, and reduce for 3 to 4 minutes, until the sauce has a syrup-like consistency.

ASSEMBLE THE DISH:

Divide the pak choi among 4 plates and place the slices of steak on top. Pour the sauce over the meat and garnish with the remaining fresh rosemary. Steamed cauliflower goes well with this dish.

Nutritional analysis per serving (175 g beef, 475 g vegetables):
calories 461, fat 29 g, saturated fat 7 g, cholesterol 62 mg, fiber 8 g, protein 37 g, carbohydrate 16 g, sodium 394 mg

BIBIMBAP-STYLE VEGETABLES WITH EGG OR TOFU IN SPICY CHILI SAUCE

Serves: 4 Prep time: 30 minutes Cook time: 20 minutes

- ½ head cauliflower, trimmed and cut into florets
- 1 courgette, sliced
- 350 g spinach
- 4 sheets nori seaweed
- 1 cucumber, sliced
- 450-g organic firm tofu or 4 omega-3 eggs
- grapeseed oil
- 2 teaspoons sesame oil
- 1 teaspoon extra virgin olive oil
- ½ tablespoon low-sodium, gluten-free tamari
- 4 tablespoons sesame seeds, lightly toasted
- 1 tablespoon chili sauce
- 1 bunch spring onions, roughly chopped
- 200 g kimchi, shop-bought or homemade (see page 311)

PREPARE THE BAP:

"Bap" means "rice". In this recipe, we'll use steamed cauliflower to create a rice-like dish. In a saucepan over a medium heat, place 1 cm water, add the cauliflower florets, cover, and let steam for 3 minutes. Drain in a colander and allow to cool. Place in a food processor and pulse until the cauliflower has a rice-like texture.

PREPARE THE VEGETABLES:

In the same way you steamed the cauliflower, lightly steam the courgette for 2 minutes so it still has crunch. Drain and set aside on a flat tray. Lightly steam the spinach in the same fashion for 2 minutes. Drain and set aside on the same tray. With kitchen scissors, cut the nori into 7.5-cm strips and set aside on the same tray. Add the sliced cucumber to them.

PREPARE THE TOFU OR EGGS:

If using tofu, slice it into pieces 5 mm thick. Heat 1 teaspoon of the sesame oil and the olive oil in a sauté pan over a medium heat. Sauté the tofu for about 3 minutes on each side until slightly golden.

If using eggs, beat them in a bowl. Heat a little grapeseed oil in a non-stick pan over a medium heat, then pour in the eggs. Cook for 2 minutes, stirring once or twice, and remove from the heat.

ASSEMBLE THE DISH:

Divide the cauliflower "rice" among 4 bowls. Arrange the vegetables on top and drizzle with tamari.

Divide the tofu or egg equally among the 4 bowls, then add the nori and sesame seeds.

Drizzle with chili sauce and the remaining sesame oil, if desired. Garnish with the spring onions and 1 to 2 tablespoons of kimchi, and serve.

Nutritional analysis per serving (1 omega-3 egg, 50 g "rice," 200 g vegetable mixture, 2 tablespoons kimchi): calories 236, fat 13 g, saturated fat 2 g, cholesterol 175 mg, fiber 5 g, protein 14 g, carbohydrate 17 g, sodium 439 mg

Nutritional analysis per serving (100 g tofu, 50 g "rice," 200 g vegetable mixture, 2 tablespoons kimchi): calories 235, fat 13 g, saturated fat 2 g, cholesterol 0 mg, fiber 6 g, protein 16 g, carbohydrate 18 g, sodium 386 mg

HOMEMADE KIMCHI

Makes: 500 to 750 g Prep time: 20 minutes, plus 48 hours maturing
- 1 head white cabbage, cored and sliced into 3- to 4-cm pieces
- 130 g coarse salt
- 5-cm piece fresh root ginger, peeled and thinly sliced
- 1 bunch spring onions, cut into 2.5-cm pieces
- 6 garlic cloves, crushed
- 40 g medium-hot dried red chili peppers, roughly ground
- optional: sliced cucumbers, daikon radish, red cabbage, turnip

Place the cabbage in a bowl, sprinkle with the salt, and allow to sit for a couple of hours. Drain off the excess liquid and stir in the remaining ingredients. Place in a large glass jar with a lid and leave in a warm place for 48 hours before serving. The kimchi will keep well in the refrigerator for up to 3 months.

Nutritional analysis per serving (60 g kimchi): calories 23, fat 0 g, saturated fat 0 g, cholesterol 0 mg, fiber 1 g, protein 2 g, carbohydrate 4 g, sodium 523 mg

CHICKEN BREAST WITH SUN-DRIED TOMATO PESTO AND SAUTÉED SPINACH

Serves: 4 Prep time: 20 minutes Cook time: 20 minutes

- 100 g sun-dried tomatoes, rinsed (see note overleaf)
- 2 garlic cloves
- 100 g raw walnuts or cashews
- salt and freshly ground black pepper, to taste
- 1 to 2 tablespoons extra virgin olive oil (see note overleaf)
- 4 boneless, skinless chicken breasts (100 to 175 g each)

SAUTÉED SPINACH:

- 1 tablespoon extra virgin olive oil
- 2 garlic cloves, crushed
- 250 g spinach
- salt and freshly ground black pepper, to taste

Preheat the oven to 180°C/Gas 4. In a food processor, combine the sun-dried tomatoes, garlic, and nuts to make a chunky pesto. Season with salt and pepper. Place the chicken breasts between cling film and lightly pound them with a meat mallet or a small, heavy-based saucepan. Make a 5-cm slit or pocket in the thicker end of each breast and stuff 1 to 2 tablespoons of the pesto into it. Secure each pocket with a toothpick (or just squeeze shut tightly).

Heat an ovenproof frying pan until medium hot. Add 1 tablespoon of the oil and sauté the chicken for 3 minutes on each side. Place the pan in the oven for about 12 minutes, or until the chicken is cooked through. Slice each breast into 3 pieces.

PREPARE THE SPINACH:

Place a pan over a medium heat and add the olive oil and garlic. Heat for 1 minute, then add the spinach. Cook just until the spinach wilts. Season with salt and pepper, then serve with the chicken.

> NOTE: Sun-dried tomatoes come either in a jar with oil, or dry. If using dry tomatoes, soak them in warm water for 5 minutes to reconstitute. Drain and discard the water and add 1 tablespoon olive oil before making the pesto. If using tomatoes soaked in olive oil, drain off the oil first; you may use this oil in the pesto.

Nutritional analysis per serving (100 g chicken, 90 g spinach):
calories 342, fat 22 g, saturated fat 3 g, cholesterol 66 mg, fiber 3 g, protein 32 g, carbohydrate 11 g, sodium 489 mg

THAI FISH SALAD

Serves: 4 Prep time: 25 minutes Cook time: 10 minutes

FISH:

- 4 snapper or bass fillets (100 to 175 g each)
- 475 ml fish stock
- 2.5-cm piece fresh root ginger, peeled and grated
- 2 tablespoons thinly sliced lemongrass

DRESSING:

- 120 ml lime juice, plus zest of 1 lime
- 2.5-cm piece fresh root ginger, peeled and grated
- 2 tablespoons low-sodium, gluten-free tamari
- ½ teaspoon green curry paste (more, if desired)
- 2 tablespoons extra virgin olive oil

SALAD:

- small handful fresh coriander leaves
- 2 garlic cloves, crushed
- 1 medium head pak choi, thinly sliced
- 1 medium carrot, peeled and thinly sliced
- 1 cucumber, peeled, seeded, and thinly sliced
- 6 asparagus spears, cut on the diagonal into 2.5-cm pieces
- 200 g bean sprouts
- 4 spring onions, sliced on the diagonal
- small handful fresh mint leaves

GARNISH:

- 1 lime, thinly sliced
- handful Thai basil leaves (any basil will work)

PREPARE THE FISH:

In an 20-cm sauté pan, place the fish in 1 cm fish stock with the ginger and lemongrass. Cover and heat slowly over a medium heat for 3 to 4 minutes, until the fish is cooked through. Remove the fish from the stock with a slotted spoon and allow it to cool on a plate.

PREPARE THE DRESSING:

Whisk all the ingredients together in a bowl or shake in a jar.

PREPARE THE SALAD:

Toss the salad ingredients in a bowl with half the dressing. Divide among 4 bowls.

ASSEMBLE THE DISH:

Place the fish on top of the salad and drizzle with the remaining dressing. Garnish with the lime slices and basil.

Nutritional analysis per serving (100 g fish, 100g salad): calories 298, fat 10 g, saturated fat 2 g, cholesterol 64 mg, fiber 4 g, protein 38 g, carbohydrate 19 g, sodium 889 mg

CHICKEN ENCRUSTED WITH RED CHILI PESTO

Serves: 4 Prep time: 30 minutes Cook time: 15 minutes

CHILI PESTO:

- 6 dried ancho chilies
- 500 to 750 ml boiling water
- 140 g raw pumpkin seeds
- 50 ml fresh lime juice
- 6 garlic cloves
- small handful fresh coriander, plus extra for garnish
- 250 ml extra virgin olive oil
- salt and freshly ground black pepper, to taste

CHICKEN:

- 1 tablespoon extra virgin olive oil or grapeseed oil
- 4 boneless, skinless chicken breasts (100 to 175 g each)
- 4 lime wedges, for garnish

PREPARE THE CHILI PESTO:

Immerse the dried chilies in boiling water until reconstituted, about 30 minutes. Drain and remove the stems and seeds. Place the chilies, pumpkin seeds, lime juice, garlic, and coriander in a food processor and blend until smooth. Slowly drizzle in the olive oil while the food processor is running, until the pesto is emulsified. Season with salt and pepper. (The pesto can be made ahead of time and stored in an airtight glass container in the refrigerator for up to 4 days. Leftover pesto is great with fresh vegetables as an afternoon snack.)

PREPARE THE CHICKEN:

Heat the olive or grapeseed oil in a sauté pan over a medium-low heat. Sauté the chicken for about 4 minutes on each side, until cooked through, or until a meat thermometer inserted in the thickest part registers at least 74°C.

ASSEMBLE THE DISH:

Heat the grill until hot. Spread about 1 tablespoon of red chili pesto over one side of each chicken breast, then grill until the pesto is crispy, 1 to 2 minutes. Garnish each plate with a lime wedge and a sprinkling of coriander. Serve with Sautéed Watercress and Spinach (see recipe below).

Nutritional analysis per serving (100 g chicken, 1 tablespoon pesto): calories 211, fat 12 g, saturated fat 2 g, cholesterol 66 mg, fiber 1 g, protein 26 g, carbohydrate 2 g, sodium 563 mg

SAUTÉED WATERCRESS AND SPINACH

Serves: 4 Prep time: 5 minutes Cook time: 5 minutes

- 1 tablespoon extra virgin olive oil
- 75 g fresh watercress
- 250 g fresh spinach
- salt, to taste

In a large sauté pan, heat the olive oil over a medium heat. Add the watercress and sauté until tender, about 3 minutes. Remove the pan from the heat and stir in the spinach to wilt. Season with salt.

Nutritional analysis per serving (180 g): calories 46, fat 4 g, saturated fat 1 g, cholesterol 0 mg, fiber 1 g, protein 2 g, carbohydrate 2 g, sodium 54 mg

GRILLED TOFU WITH CORIANDER PESTO

Serves: 4 Prep time: 15 minutes Cook time: 10 minutes

- 3 tablespoons low-sodium, gluten-free tamari
- 2 tablespoons sesame oil
- 475 ml organic firm tofu, cut into 8 slices
- 2 medium courgettes, sliced on the diagonal into 5-mm slices
- 90 g fresh basil
- 2 garlic cloves, chopped
- 1-cm piece fresh root ginger, peeled and chopped
- 3 spring onions, chopped
- 35 g raw pine nuts or walnuts

- 120 ml extra virgin olive oil (reserve 1 tablespoon)
- salt and freshly ground black pepper, to taste
- 100 g rocket or other salad greens

PREPARE THE TOFU AND COURGETTES:

Combine the tamari and sesame oil in a shallow bowl. Place the tofu slices and courgettes in the bowl and marinate for 10 minutes. Heat a grill or griddle pan until medium hot, then cook the courgettes first, about 2 minutes on each side. Set aside. Cook the tofu for about 3 minutes on each side and set aside.

PREPARE THE PESTO:

Combine the basil, garlic, ginger, spring onions, nuts, and most of the olive oil in a food processor and pulse until smooth. If the consistency is too thick, thin it with a little water. Season with salt and pepper.

ASSEMBLE THE DISH:

Toss the rocket or other salad greens with the reserved tablespoon of olive oil and divide among 4 plates. Arrange the tofu and courgettes on top and drizzle with the pesto.

Nutritional analysis per serving (2 slices tofu, ¼ courgette): calories 458, fat 25 g, saturated fat 6 g, cholesterol 0 mg, fiber 4 g, protein 15 g, carbohydrate 10 g, sodium 549 mg

DIPS AND SPREADS

HOMEMADE OLIVE TAPENADE

Makes: 200 g Prep time: 5 minutes

- 350 g stoned Kalamata olives
- 3 garlic cloves
- 250 ml extra virgin olive oil
- small handful fresh parsley, chopped

- 1 teaspoon chopped fresh thyme
- 1 teaspoon chopped fresh rosemary
- zest of 1 lemon, plus juice of ½ lemon
- freshly ground black pepper, to taste

Place all the ingredients in a food processor and process for about 2 minutes. Store in an airtight container in the refrigerator for up to 5 days.

Nutritional analysis per serving (60 g): calories 172, fat 19 g, saturated fat 3 g, cholesterol 0 mg, fiber 1 g, protein 0 g, carbohydrate 1 g, sodium 197 mg

TAHINI DIPPING SAUCE

Makes: 150 g Prep time: 5 minutes
- 115 g tahini (sesame seed paste, preferably raw)
- 1 garlic clove
- 120 ml extra virgin olive oil
- 120 ml water
- juice of 1 lemon
- salt, to taste
- optional: 2 tablespoons finely chopped fresh dill

Blend all the ingredients in a blender for about 2 minutes, until smooth. Store in an airtight container in the refrigerator for up to 5 days.

Nutritional analysis per serving (2 tablespoons): calories 191, fat 21 g, saturated fat 3 g, cholesterol 0 mg, fiber 1 g, protein 1 g, carbohydrate 2 g, sodium 107 mg

SPINACH AND WALNUT PESTO

Makes: 375 to 500 g Prep time: 5 minutes
- 60 to 90 g spinach
- 30 g fresh basil leaves
- handful fresh parsley
- 65 g raw walnuts or pine nuts
- 50 ml extra virgin olive oil

- ½ teaspoon salt
- 1 garlic clove

Place all the ingredients in a food processor and pulse to a slightly chunky consistency. Store in an airtight container in the refrigerator for up to 5 days.

Nutritional analysis per serving (2 tablespoons): calories 107, fat 11 g, saturated fat 1 g, cholesterol 0 mg, fiber 1 g, protein 2 g, carbohydrate 2 g, sodium 156 mg

SUN-DRIED TOMATO DIP

Makes: 375 ml Prep time: 10 minutes

- 1 medium-to-large fresh tomato, cut into chunks
- 50 g sun-dried tomatoes, diced (see note below)
- 1 garlic clove
- 1 tablespoon chopped fresh parsley
- 50 ml extra virgin olive oil
- 1 tablespoon raw pine nuts
- ½ teaspoon salt
- ½ teaspoon freshly ground black pepper

Blend all the ingredients in a blender until smooth, about 2 minutes. Add more salt and pepper to taste. Store in an airtight container in the refrigerator for up to 5 days.

NOTE: Sun-dried tomatoes come either in a jar with oil or dry. If using dry tomatoes, soak them in warm water for 5 minutes to reconstitute. Drain and discard the water and add 1 tablespoon olive oil before making the pesto. If using tomatoes soaked in olive oil, drain off the oil first; you may use it in the pesto.

Nutritional analysis per serving (50 ml): calories 126, fat 9 g, saturated fat 1 g, cholesterol 0 mg, fiber 3 g, protein 3 g, carbohydrate 9 g, sodium 209 mg

Miso Dipping Sauce

Makes: 375 ml Prep time: 10 minutes

- 3 tablespoons gluten- and wheat-free white or red miso paste
- 120 ml extra virgin olive oil
- juice of ½ lemon
- 1 garlic clove
- 120 ml water
- 1 tablespoon cider vinegar
- 1 tablespoon low-sodium, gluten-free tamari
- 2.5-cm piece fresh root ginger, peeled

Blend all the ingredients in a food processor until smooth, about 2 minutes. Store in an airtight jar in the refrigerator for up to 5 days.

Nutritional analysis per serving (50 ml): calories 99, fat 10 g, saturated fat 1 g, cholesterol 0 mg, fiber 0 g, protein 0 g, carbohydrate 2 g, sodium 233 mg

Resources

At www.10daydetox.com/resources, you will find all the resources listed below, and more, for support during and long after the Blood Sugar Solution 10-Day Detox.

Health and Testing Resources

Basic lab testing guidelines

The Blood Sugar Solution Diabesity Quiz

The *How to Work with Your Doctor to Get What You Need* downloadable guide

Testing tools (including glucose monitors, FitBit Wi-Fi Smart Scale or Withings scale, blood pressure monitors, and personal movement trackers)

Symptoms Tracking Chart (to test gluten and dairy)

The 10-Day Detox Online Health Tracker

The 10-Day Detox supplements

10-Day Detox Community Resources

The 10-Day Detox Online Course

The 10-Day Detox Online Community

How to lead a 10-Day Detox Group

How to find a local food co-op

Life coaching resources

Lifestyle Resources

Fitness resources

The *UltraCalm* guided relaxation program

Meditation resources

Herbal resources

Stress-busting tools

Food

Brand recommendations for 10-Day Detox Staples Shopping List

Brand recommendations for Emergency Life Pack

The *Restaurant Rescue Guide*

Other Resources

I encourage you to explore my website, www.drhyman.com for more articles, videos, and guidance on how to create health and well-being.

I also encourage you to get a copy of *The Blood Sugar Solution* and *The Blood Sugar Solution Cookbook* (www.bloodsugarsolution.com). These will help you transition from the 10-Day Detox to build a plan for long-term health.

Acknowledgments

This is a book I wish I didn't feel compelled to write. Facing the reality of food addiction is tough. But seeing how many suffer needlessly from the prison of food addiction, and witnessing how many of my patients were able to quickly overcome it by applying simple scientific principles that most don't know, I knew I had to write this book.

I am grateful to all the scientists who work tirelessly to dissect the biology of how food affects us, particularly two friends, David Ludwig, MD, of Harvard, and Kelly Brownell, PhD, of Yale. They are dedicated scientists who have broken tough ground to call attention to this issue and to prove the science behind it. Read their work; it is revolutionary.

I thank my patients who trusted me to translate that science into practical strategies for their healing. They have shown me through their struggles and success exactly how real this problem is, and how easily it can be solved with the right approach.

Words cannot adequately express my gratitude for my agent, Richard Pine, who has guided me and gently pushed me to speak what is true. A big thank-you to Tracy Behar, my editor, and all my friends and supporters at Little, Brown, who saw the possibility of a new solution to our health care crisis and created a fabulous home for the ideas of functional medicine. And to Debra Goldstein, who helped me shape, massage, and craft this manuscript with love and passion, thank you. The jukebox is always on!

A special thanks to my UltraTeam: Anne McLaughlin, Kate

Johnson, Gerry Doherty, Shibani Subramanya, Daffnee Cohen, Robert Oakes, and Lizzy Swick, who make it possible for me to do the work I love every day.

My thanks extend to many more who have inspired, helped, and supported me. The list would be too long if I named everyone individually, but you know who you are—thank you, thank you, thank you. I must mention a few special people: Jeffrey Bland, who cracked open my world twelve years ago (and it has never been the same); my friends and cofaculty and board members at the Institute for Functional Medicine, Laurie Hoffman, David Jones, Patrick Hanaway, Kristi Hughes, Dan Lukazker, and the many others who make it happen.

To my cocreators and fellow medical and wellness activists who have inspired me and continue to create seismic shifts in our way of thinking and living, thank you: Dean Ornish, Mehmet C. Oz, James Gordon, Andrew Weil, Deepak Chopra, Christiane Northrup, Daniel and Tara Goleman, Jon Kabat-Zinn, Leo Galland, Sidney Baker, David Perlmutter, Frank Lipman, Patrick Hanaway, Robert Hedaya, Joel Evans, David Eisenberg, Bethany Hayes, David Jones, Tracy Gaudet, Kenneth Pelletier, Peter Libby, and Martha Herbert. A special thanks to Arianna Huffington for providing a place for the truth to be told. Thank you, Rick Warren, Dee Eastman, and all my friends at Saddleback for believing that we can all get healthy together.

Without the support of my team at the UltraWellness Center, where I do my primary work of seeing patients, I couldn't begin to do anything else. You are my foundation and at the core of my life. Your contributions wash over me daily. Thank you for showing up and believing.

My friends and partners at the Handel Group—Lauren Zander, Joe Seibert, Erik Van Dillen, Katie Torpey, Amy Teuteberg, Andy Youmans, and others—help me dream the dream and make transformation happen. I thank you beyond measure!!

Most importantly, my family has supported me in my crazy passion for changing the way we practice medicine and creating a healthier world for all of us. I could not have done this without all your love and belief in what I am doing. Thank you, Rachel, Misha, Ruth, Saul, Jesse, Ben, Sarah, Paul, Lauren, Jake, and Zachary. It is for you and because of you that I wake up every day grateful and joyful.

And to Pilar Gerasimo, my co–health revolutionary and partner, who chewed over every word and made this book speak loudly for all. Thank you for your genius and your love!

Lastly, a profound thank-you goes out to all those who participated in the trial run of the Blood Sugar Solution 10-Day Detox Diet and showed just how powerful food can be to heal and renew.

General Index

Advanced Plan, 211, 220–21
Adventure Plan
  features of, 11
  goal of, 66–67, 253
  meals and snacks, 120
advertising, 23–24, 25, 241
Ahmed, Serge H., 29
alcohol, 76, 81, 97, 105, 106, 231
allergies, 58, 77, 78, 88, 214, 215
Amen, Daniel, 68–69
Ames, Bruce, 32–33
antioxidants, 84–85
appetite controls, 30, 31, 32, 36, 40–41, 57, 88
apps
  for stress release, 179
  tracking results with, 198–99
artificial sweeteners, 8, 34–36, 75, 79, 85, 98, 224

Basic Supplement Pack, 101
beans/legumes
  Advanced Plan and, 220
  Basic Plan and, 223
  Blood Sugar Solution Plan for Life and, 226
  elimination of, 76, 79, 87, 99
  protein paired with, 222
bedroom, as sanctuary, 124, 186–87
behavior
  food addiction and, 27–29, 36–37
  low-friction behavior change, 184
behavior design, 184
belly fat, 3–4, 30–31, 41, 44, 51, 56, 85–86, 91, 175
biology
  food addiction and, 29–31, 37, 47
  genetics and, 43–46
  resetting, 60
biomarkers, 50
blood pressure, 12, 70, 74, 109, 218
blood pressure monitor, 104, 109
blood sugar
  balancing, 3, 4, 12, 70, 75, 84, 87–88, 102, 108

caffeine and, 82
exercise and, 88
food addiction and, 18–19
medications for, 12, 74
testing yourself, 72
Blood Sugar Solution 10-Day Detox Community, 248
Blood Sugar Solution 10-Day Detox Diet. *See also* Prep Phase; 10-Day Detox Phase; Transition Phase
  community support for, 12, 67–70
  as disruptive, 39
  eating guidelines, 64–67
  exercise and, 51
  in with the good, 83–93
  high-impact changes and, 54, 55
  lifestyle practices, 60, 75, 83–84, 132
  as long-term fix, 59–60
  online 10-Day Detox Diet Course, 11, 12, 70, 109, 202, 204, 205
  out with the bad, 75–83
  rationale for, 8–9
  scientific basis of, 56–60
  tracking results, 71–72
  transition programs, 55
  weight loss and, 3, 9, 70–71
The Blood Sugar Solution Cookbook (Hyman), 185, 219, 221, 223, 225, 231, 247
Blood Sugar Solution for Life, 212
The Blood Sugar Solution (Hyman), 3, 25, 55, 64, 214, 220, 222, 242
Blood Sugar Solution Plan for Life, 224–31
Bloomberg, Michael, 238
BMI (body mass index), 48, 70
bowel movements. *See also* gut function
  detoxification symptoms and, 140
  emptying and, 143–44
  hydration and, 90, 144
  strategies for easy elimination, 144–45
  supplements and, 102, 103–04, 118, 145

Recipe Index

Recipe Index

About the Author

Mark Hyman, MD, believes that we all deserve a life of vitality—and that we have the potential to create it for ourselves. That's why he is dedicated to tackling the root causes of chronic disease by harnessing the power of functional medicine to transform healthcare. Dr. Hyman and his team work every day to empower people, organizations, and communities to heal their bodies and minds, and improve our social and economic resilience.

Dr. Hyman is a practicing family physician, a six-time #1 *New York Times* bestselling author, and an internationally recognized leader, speaker, educator, and advocate in his field. He is also the founder and medical director of the UltraWellness Center, chairman of the board of the Institute for Functional Medicine, a medical editor of the *Huffington Post,* and a regular medical contributor on Katie Couric's TV show, *Katie.*

Dr. Hyman works with individuals and organizations, as well as policy makers and influencers. He has testified before both the White House Commission on Complementary and Alternative Medicine and the Senate Working Group on Health Care Reform on Functional Medicine. He has consulted with the Surgeon General on diabetes prevention and participated in the 2009 White House Forum on Prevention and Wellness. Senator Tom Harkin of Iowa nominated Dr. Hyman for the President's Advisory Group on Prevention, Health Promotion, and Integrative and Public Health. In addition, Dr. Hyman has worked with President Clinton, presenting at the Clinton Foundation's Health Matters, Achieving Wellness in Every Generation conference, and the Clinton Global Initiative, as well as with the World Economic Forum on global health issues.

Dr. Hyman also works with fellow leaders in his field to help people and communities thrive—with Rick Warren, Dr. Mehmet Oz, and Dr. Daniel Amen, he created the Daniel Plan, a faith-based initiative that helped the Saddleback Church collectively lose 250,000 pounds (113,000 kg). He has appeared as an advisor on *The Dr. Oz Show* and is on the board of Dr. Oz's HealthCorps, which tackles the obesity epidemic by educating American students about nutrition. With Dr. Dean Ornish and Dr. Michael Roizen, Dr. Hyman crafted and helped introduce the Take Back Your Health Act of 2009 to the United States Senate to provide for reimbursement of lifestyle treatment of chronic disease.

Join Dr. Hyman on his path to revolutionize the way we think about and take care of our health and our societies at www.drhyman.com, on Twitter and Instagram @markhymanmd, and on Facebook at facebook.com/drmarkhyman.